Dr David Cavan is an internationally renowned consultant endocrinologist with expertise in all areas of diabetes and weight management. He specialises in supporting people to make lifestyle changes to manage and reverse Type 2 diabetes and using weight loss injections where appropriate, in helping people lose weight and improve health. Further information is available at www.thediabetesdoctor.co.uk.

Also by Dr David Cavan:

How to Reverse Type 2 Diabetes and Prediabetes

Reverse your Diabetes Diet

Take Control of Type 1 Diabetes

The Low-Carb Diabetes Cookbook

Managing Type 2 Diabetes

A Guide to Weight-Loss Injections

*How to maximise weight loss,
minimise side effects – and keep the weight off*

Dr David Cavan

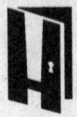

The information in this book may not be suitable for everyone and is not intended to be a substitute for medical advice or medical treatment. You are advised to consult a doctor on any matters relating to your health, and in particular on any matters that may require diagnosis or medical attention. Any use of the information in this book is made on the reader's good judgement after consulting with his or her doctor and is the reader's sole responsibility.

Copyright © Dr David Cavan 2026

The right of Dr David Cavan to be identified as the Author of the Work has been asserted by him in accordance with the Copyright, Designs and Patents Act 1988.

First published in 2026 by Headline Home
an imprint of Headline Publishing Group Limited

1

Apart from any use permitted under UK copyright law, this publication may only be reproduced, stored, or transmitted, in any form, or by any means, with prior permission in writing of the publishers or, in the case of reprographic production, in accordance with the terms of licences issued by the Copyright Licensing Agency.

Every effort has been made to fulfil requirements with regard to reproducing copyright material. The author and publisher will be glad to rectify any omissions at the earliest opportunity.

Cataloguing in Publication Data is available from the British Library

Paperback ISBN 978 1 0354 3042 0
eISBN 978 1 0354 3043 7

Typeset in Dante by CC Book Production
Printed and bound in Great Britain by Clays Ltd, Elcograf S.p.A.

Headline's policy is to use papers that are natural, renewable and recyclable products and made from wood grown in well-managed forests and other controlled sources. The logging and manufacturing processes are expected to conform to the environmental regulations of the country of origin.

Headline Publishing Group Limited
An Hachette UK Company
Carmelite House
50 Victoria Embankment
London
EC4Y 0DZ

The authorised representative in the EEA is Hachette Ireland,
8 Castlecourt Centre, Dublin 15, D15 XTP3, Ireland
(email: info@hbgi.ie)

www.headline.co.uk
www.hachette.co.uk

Contents

	Introduction	1
1.	A history of obesity and weight-loss treatments	9
2.	What is Obesity?	19
3.	Eating for success on weight-loss injections	51
4.	What kinds of exercise should I do while on weight-loss injections?	85
5.	Wegovy and Mounjaro	101
6.	Other benefits of weight-loss injections	115
7.	Side effects of weight-loss injections and how to manage them	127
8.	How can I maximise the effect, and minimise the side effects, of weight-loss injections?	145
9.	Starting injections – and staying the course	165

10.	The importance of managing stress, mood and sleep while on weight-loss injections	181
11.	Successfully coming off injections	199
12.	Life after injections	211
13.	Future developments	223
	Index	233

Introduction

I have been a hospital consultant specialising in diabetes for almost thirty years. Over that time I have watched in horror as rates of obesity have skyrocketed in the UK, leading to an epidemic of Type 2 diabetes. From 2013–16 I was the Director of Policy at the International Diabetes Federation, which opened my eyes to the devastating effects of obesity across the globe. During my career I have seen several medications introduced to help people lose weight. Many came with great promise, but most have since been withdrawn due to serious side effects. None had the impact of the new drugs that are the subject of this book. Rarely has a group of drugs made headlines like the weight-loss injections (WLIs) – such as Wegovy, Ozempic and Mounjaro – have. At the time of writing (October 2025), barely a week goes by without a press article about the effects of these drugs, both good and bad, on individuals or on the human race. It is encouraging that the problem of increased obesity in our population is getting wider coverage, and while these injections can certainly help, they are not in themselves the answer to any one individual's health problem or to a healthy future for humanity.

But what a turnaround. Throughout history, humankind has had to endure hunger and, at times, famine. While in modern times we generally associate famine with crop failures in Africa, widespread famines occurred in Ukraine and other Soviet republics in the 1920s–1940s, in Cambodia in the 1970s and North Korea in the 1990s. Closer to home, the potato famine in Ireland in the 1840s led to an estimated million deaths. Thankfully, advances in agriculture and food production have ensured a more reliable food supply in Europe and many other parts of the world, so that widespread famine in the traditional sense of the word no longer occurs. However, there is a downside to this: largely unchecked, the food industry has been able to produce highly processed products (I refuse to call them foods) that are cheap, high in calories and low in nutrition. This has led to a new type of malnutrition, characterised not by weight loss and starvation but by weight gain, obesity and, paradoxically, hunger. At an individual level, this leads to eating more of the same products and a vicious cycle of more weight gain and a whole host of conditions associated with obesity and metabolic ill health – Type 2 diabetes, high blood pressure, dementia, some cancers, heart disease and strokes. In the UK, obesity-related illnesses cost the National Health Service

(NHS) £11 billion a year. And all the while, the food industry gets richer and richer.

Of course, the ideal response to this scenario would be to reform our food environment, and for governments to use their huge powers to discourage the production of ultra-processed foods and encourage the consumption of nutritious, real foods. But so far, with a few notable exceptions, that is not happening. Instead, the pharmaceutical industry has come up with medications to undo the harmful effects of the food industry's products. Now, given the current situation, with record levels of obesity in our population, these drugs have a valid place. They play a role in helping those who are most severely affected, and who can tolerate taking them, to lose weight. However, unlike simplistic interpretations of policymakers' announcements such as how 'weight-loss jabs could help the unemployed get back to work', they need to be seen as just one part of the solution, not the whole solution.

In the UK, the use of these drugs is governed by guidelines from the National Institute for Health and Care Excellence (NICE), which state that, when taken for weight loss, Wegovy can only be prescribed to people with obesity within a specialist weight management service that provides multidisciplinary care. Mounjaro can also be prescribed by GPs, but they are also expected to provide 'wraparound care'. That means not just prescribing the medication, but also providing advice on diet and physical activity and, where appropriate, addressing the psychological factors that affect food choices. It also means advising patients about, and monitoring for, side effects. So far, so good – that is exactly the context in which I believe that weight-loss injections should be used. The problem is that while these services do exist in many areas of the country, their limited capacity means they can only scratch the surface of the obesity epidemic sweeping across the UK and much of the rest of the world. As a result, many people are turning to online services where, after a brief 'consultation' based on answering a questionnaire, and paying around £150, they are sent their first doses of the drug in the post, with no supervision or meaningful follow-up. Some people do really well following this route. Others do less well, and feature in horror stories in the press about the side effects of weight-loss injections.

The most common side effects affect the gut, and include nausea, vomiting, heartburn, diarrhoea and constipation. Headache, tiredness and dizziness are also listed, although these can occur with many different types of medication. Often these side effects settle down as your system gets used to the medication, but sometimes the symptoms persist or even get worse. More serious side effects include gallstones, a type of paralysis of the stomach called gastroparesis, and inflammation of the pancreas (pancreatitis) that can lead to a stay in intensive care. In animal studies the drugs have been linked to cancer of the thyroid gland. There is also data suggesting that they cause disproportionate loss of muscle mass, which can lead to more health problems. We do not yet know the effects of being on these drugs continuously for years, and so some experts recommend that treatment be limited to two years – which is also my approach. It is therefore important that everyone who takes one of these medications understands how they work, the benefits of taking them, and the drawbacks. In this book I share a number of tips on how to get these drugs to work better for you, how to minimise side effects, and how to retrain your appetite towards foods that will naturally keep you fuller for longer, so that when you come off the medication you do not go back to your old eating habits, which led you to being overweight in the first place.

These weight-loss drugs were originally developed as treatments for people with Type 2 diabetes. This is a condition in which the body becomes resistant to the effect of the hormone insulin, leading to higher than normal levels of glucose in the blood. Unlike almost all other diabetes treatments, these drugs were not only effective in reducing blood glucose levels, but they also helped people lose weight. That led to further refinements to develop drugs that were particularly effective at weight loss, and to the release of Saxenda, Wegovy and Mounjaro specifically for weight loss. Saxenda has to be taken once daily and is less commonly used now.

Dr David Cavan

In this book, we focus on Wegovy and Mounjaro. For people who are obese and have Type 2 diabetes, these drugs will help both conditions. Since so many other problems are related to obesity and metabolic ill health, it is not surprising that these drugs can also help other conditions, and this book discusses in detail the evidence that they can help people with heart disease, kidney disease, high blood pressure, sleep apnoea and polycystic ovary syndrome, and can also help reduce the risk of dementia. We will also look at the intriguing evidence showing how they can be used to curb not just 'normal' food cravings, but excessive cravings that lead to binge eating or even binge drinking.

This book is for anyone who is affected by obesity and who wants to do something about it. It discusses what obesity is, how it comes about, and how these medications can be part of the solution. However, it is not just for people who want to use weight-loss injections, as it provides valuable information to people who want to have a go (or another go) at changing their lifestyle as the first step in losing weight. Many weight management services require this as a precursor to starting injections, and this is the approach I recommend.

This book is also not just for people with obesity, but for their loved ones and carers too. In my experience, someone who has the support and understanding of their spouse or other family members, especially those who do the household food shop or cook their meals, is far more likely to be able to sustain lifestyle changes in the longer term, which will be essential for when the WLI treatment comes to an end.

This book is – of course – for anyone who is thinking about, or who is already taking, weight-loss injections. It provides detailed information about how the injections work, as well as practical information about how to take them and how to minimise side effects. We will discuss how you can access them via the NHS or privately, and provide step-by-step advice on how to take the medications. The book explains how other conditions can be affected by the injections, and whether – and how – to adjust other medications you take.

It examines how you can increase the effect of these medications by choosing foods that naturally increase your body's production of GLP-1 (the hormone activated by the drugs), and how to change your eating habits while you are taking the injections, so you can come off the injections successfully – without regaining weight. Above all, my aim is that this book provides a practical guide to navigating your weight-loss journey before, during and after your treatment with weight-loss injections.

Chapter 1

A history of obesity and weight-loss treatments

For most of human history, obesity was rare for our species. In fact, as civilisations emerged, carrying excess weight had positive connotations, as it was associated with being wealthy and powerful. In medieval art, beautiful women were typically painted or sculpted with figures we would describe as overweight. King Henry VIII was morbidly obese and reportedly had a 54-inch waist. Some of the early US presidents were obese at a time when it was considered a symbol of prosperity and strength, even health. William Taft, who was president from 1909 to 1913, reportedly weighed 340 pounds (154 kilograms) and had a body mass index of 45, indicative of severe obesity. He suffered from some of the consequences of obesity, including sleep apnoea.[1]

From the mid-1800s, however, obesity was recognised as being associated with ill health, particularly Type 2 diabetes,

---

[1] Rudolph M (1960), *The Health of Presidents*. New York: Putnam.

and by the early 1900s evidence began to emerge from the insurance industry that excess weight was associated with increased mortality. Nevertheless, ingrained attitudes are slow to give way, and since being thin had long been associated with poverty – and its dreadful accompaniments malnutrition and disease – the notion that carrying extra weight was healthy persisted well into the twentieth century.

By the end of the twentieth century, obesity rates had begun to soar, initially in richer societies such as the USA and later across the globe. With increasing rates of obesity came many other health problems, and for the first time in history humans had a new problem: they had to lose, rather than gain, weight. Public perceptions of obesity had also changed, and people with obesity were stigmatised and criticised for their weight. Being slim was healthy – and fashionable.

The relationship between food and obesity was first identified in the 1700s. In 1797, the Scottish military surgeon John Rollo found that a diet low in carbohydrate helped people with diabetes lose weight, and in 1863 William Banting, an English undertaker, published 'Letter on Corpulence', detailing his personal struggles with obesity and his weight-loss success with a low-carbohydrate diet.[2] Many types of diet have been

---

[2] Banting W. 'Letter on corpulence, addressed to the public.' *Obesity Res.*, 1993, 1: 153–63.

invented over the years, but Banting's approach is one of the most successful, and has been copied by many other diets, such as Atkins and keto. Changing one's diet is notoriously difficult, as it means changing lifelong habits, and it is not entirely surprising that over the years, people have turned to their doctors for medication to help them lose weight.

People with high levels of thyroid hormone (thyrotoxicosis) lose weight because the thyroid hormone increases the body's metabolic rate. One of the earliest medical approaches to weight loss was the use of thyroid extract in the late nineteenth century. However, the human body is very sensitive to small changes in levels of thyroid hormone, and the high level necessary for weight loss also causes several less beneficial effects. These include a rapid heart rate, anxiety, confusion and, over time, heart failure and osteoporosis. Some unlicensed weight-loss products today include thyroid hormones, and these are best avoided because of these adverse effects.

One of the more bizarre approaches was the use of pills containing the eggs of tapeworms. The theory was that tapeworms would develop in the gut and absorb the person's food, leading to weight loss. Needless to say, this approach is risky, as tapeworms can also find their way into the brain and can cause epilepsy, meningitis and dementia.

Developed in the 1920s, amphetamines were one of the first medications used to promote weight loss. These are stimulant drugs that work by increasing the levels of dopamine, norepinephrine and serotonin in the brain. These are neurotransmitters that send signals between cells in the brain, and so amphetamines cause increased activity in the brain. The increase in dopamine leads to a decrease in appetite. Amphetamines also increase the heart rate and breathing rate, thus increasing the energy used by the body and leading to weight loss. Yet again, several side effects are observed when using amphetamines, including anxiety and difficulty sleeping. More severe side effects include depression and other mental health issues, abnormal heart rhythms, heart attack and stroke. They are also highly addictive.

The weight-loss effects of amphetamines led to the development of medications such as fenfluramine and dexfenfluramine that specifically increase serotonin levels. They were used for a period in the 1990s, but were later withdrawn because of heart and lung complications. Sibutramine was a similar drug, withdrawn in 2010 because of an increased risk of heart attack and stroke. Human nature being what it is, unscrupulous producers have continued to include sibutramine in diet supplements. Rimonabant works by blocking cannabinoid receptors in the brain to reduce appetite. It was withdrawn in 2008 because of an increase in depression and other psychiatric disorders.

A Guide to Weight Loss Injections

Orlistat was developed in the 1990s as a treatment for obesity, by working in the gut rather than the brain. It prevents the absorption of fat from the gut into the bloodstream. But as the fat stays in the gut, it causes the stools to become loose and oily (known as steatorrhoea) if fat is eaten. It is therefore designed to encourage a low-fat diet. But thanks to research carried out over the past twenty years, scientists realised that fat is not the enemy we once thought it was, and that reducing carbohydrates is likely to be a more effective weight-loss approach; orlistat generally has quite a modest effect on weight loss. Unlike many of the other weight-loss medications, it is still available and in many countries it can be purchased without a prescription.

In summary, the track record of weight-loss medications through the ages is not a good one, with most being taken off the market after it was proven that they caused more harm than good. I can be forgiven, then, for feeling rather sceptical when Byetta, the first of a brand-new class of drugs called GLP-1 agonists, appeared on the scene in 2007. Byetta was a treatment for Type 2 diabetes rather than a weight-loss drug, but it came with evidence from research studies that showed that not only did it help reduce glucose levels in people with diabetes, but it also helped them lose weight – and sometimes a lot of weight. The problem was that it had to be given by injection twice a day. While some people seemed to do very well on Byetta, over time I noticed that many did not lose much weight. I suspect this was because having an injection twice a day was quite a big ask, and they missed some or all of their injections. Yet, this was the start of the journey that was to lead to the development of Wegovy and Mounjaro, today's weight-loss injections.

The story starts in the 1980s, when scientists were trying to gain a better understanding of duodenal ulcer disease. In the past, many people had to undergo surgery to remove parts of the gut because of ulcer disease. Thanks to modern medicines that treat ulcers in the very early stages, ulcers are generally no longer a cause of serious gut haemorrhage or death and surgical treatments are now thankfully obsolete. As part of his research into ulcer medications, Professor Jens Juul Holst from Copenhagen, Denmark, was looking into the potential role of a newly discovered molecule, GLP-1 (glucagon-like peptide 1). He found that when GLP-1 was pumped through pig pancreases, it increased the production of insulin, the hormone responsible for regulating glucose levels in the blood. He also found that it reduced the production of glucagon, which increases glucose levels, by the pancreas. These effects alone would be crucial in treating people with Type 2 diabetes. Once early trials started in people, another big effect was noticed: that GLP-1 significantly reduced appetite. Since many people with Type 2 diabetes are overweight, it added a third important dimension to the potential of GLP-1 as a treatment.

Subsequent research has found that GLP-1 has many different effects. Its effect on increasing insulin production in the pancreas has been shown only to occur after the person has eaten. This is important as it means that, unlike insulin injections, which can cause glucose levels to go too low, GLP-1 only increases insulin release when it is needed: that is, when the blood glucose level rises after eating. GLP-1 also ensures that the pancreas's store of insulin is always kept full, by promoting the development of insulin-producing beta cells. GLP-1 slows down the contractions of the stomach, so that food stays in the stomach longer before going into the small intestine. This fullness increases satiety (the feeling of being full) after meals and reduces the desire for more food. GLP-1 also has effects in the brain to increase satiety and reduce appetite.[3]

The problem was that GLP-1 only lasts in the circulation for a few minutes, and so a lot of research and development over many years was required to produce a drug that could increase GLP-1 levels for longer. The solution to this challenge came in an unlikely form – the Gila monster, a species of venomous lizard native to south-western USA and north-western Mexico. It is a heavy, slow-moving reptile up to

---

3 Holst JJ, 'From the incretin concept and the discovery of GKP-1 to today's diabetes therapy.' *Front. Endocrinol.*, 2019, 10: 260. doi:10.3389/fendo.2019.00260

22 inches (56 centimetres) long. Its bite causes such extreme pain that it led curious scientists to study its saliva, trying to identify what it contained. They discovered that one of its components is a hormone known as Exendin-4, which was found to have similar effects as GLP-1.[4] Byetta contains the drug exenatide, which is a synthetic version of Exendin-4. Byetta works by mimicking the effects of GLP-1: increasing insulin secretion, reducing glucagon, increasing satiety and reducing appetite. As well as reducing glucose levels in people with diabetes, it also played a role in helping people reduce weight. Researchers then developed newer drugs that had a bigger impact on weight loss and that only had to be given once a week – a big step forward from the twice-daily injections required for Byetta. The most potent GLP-1 drug is semaglutide, the active ingredient of Wegovy and Ozempic.

Mounjaro also increases GLP-1 actions – but with a difference. It also increases the impact of gastric inhibitory polypeptide (GIP), which increases the secretion of insulin, reducing glucagon and slowing the emptying of the stomach.

After many false starts with different weight-loss medications that have come and gone, we now have drugs that offer real hope to people who have struggled with obesity for many

---

[4] Furman B, 'The development of Byetta (exenatide) from the venom of the Gila monster as an antidiabetic agent.' *Toxicon.*, 2012, 59: 464–71.

years, but they have their downsides, as do all medications. In this book we will explore these drugs in detail, to give you clear advice about how they work, who can and cannot take them, what they can – and cannot – do, and what you can do to help them work most effectively on your weight-loss journey.

Chapter 2
What is obesity?

Obesity means having too much body fat, and this increases the risk of various health problems. It is typically measured using the body mass index (BMI), which expresses the relationship between a person's height and their weight. Normal body weight is defined as a BMI between 20 and 25. A BMI less than 20 is suggestive that a person is underweight, while a BMI of 25–30 is defined as overweight, and above 30 as obese. To find your BMI, you take your weight in kilograms and divide it by the square of your height in metres. So, for a person who weighs 80 kilos (about 176 pounds) and is 1.83 m tall (about 6 feet), their BMI is calculated as $80/(1.83 \times 1.83) = 23.9$ (which is in the normal range).

A person of the same height who weighs 110 kilos (about 240 pounds) has a BMI of $110/(1.83 \times 1.83) = 32.9$ (which is in the obese range). You can work out your BMI on the NHS website.

BMI is generally not used for children, and care must be taken when dealing with individuals who are very muscular. Muscle weighs more than fat, and it is quite possible for someone to be 'overweight', according to their BMI, but to be perfectly fit and healthy; their 'excess' body weight is because of large muscles. For this reason it has been suggested that waist circumference is a better indicator of obesity, as most people who are overweight because of excess fat have large fat stores around their middle. As a general rule, if your waist measures over half your height you are likely to be carrying excess fat. Do not use your trouser size as a waist measurement. Instead, pass a tape measure around your waist at the level of your belly button, where many of us are at our widest. So if you are 1.7 m tall (about 5 ft 8 in), your waist should be no more than half of this (85 cm or 34 in).

Because of the limitations of BMI to define obesity, in 2025 the medical journal *Lancet Diabetes and Endocrinology* published a paper on the work of a global panel of experts who had reviewed the definition of obesity.[5] The experts proposed that people with a BMI above 30 be classified into one of three groups:

---

[5] Rubino F, et al. 'Definition and diagnostic criteria of clinical obesity.' *Lancet Diabetes and Endocrinology*, 2025. https://doi.org/10.1016/S2213-8587(24)00316-4

A Guide to Weight Loss Injections

- *No obesity.* People who do not have excess body fat, but whose BMI is high because of high muscle mass. They will generally not have an increased waist circumference.
- *Preclinical obesity.* People who have excess body fat (and increased waist circumference) but who are otherwise healthy.
- *Clinical obesity.* People with excess body fat who have health problems related to their obesity.

So, what does this mean in practice? People with no obesity are generally healthy and, as they do not have increased body fat, have no need for any type of treatment to lose weight. Their high BMI is a result of high muscle mass, which is a good thing!

People with preclinical obesity are, by definition, healthy, with no evidence that their excess body weight is causing any health problems. However, over time their body weight could cause problems, such as arthritis or sleep apnoea, and they would likely benefit from losing weight to reduce the likelihood of such problems occurring.

People with clinical obesity are unhealthy. The *Lancet* definition states that they either have evidence of reduced organ or tissue function due to obesity (for example, Type 2 diabetes, heart disease, fatty liver disease), or their daily activities are severely limited, reflecting the effect of obesity on mobility or basic activities of daily living (for example, because of joint problems or shortness of breath). The *Lancet* recommends that people with clinical obesity should receive timely, evidence-based treatment, with the aim to induce improvement (or remission, when possible) of the clinical manifestations of obesity, and prevent progression to organ damage.

This new definition makes sense, and does not lump everyone into the same category based purely on their BMI. It correctly implies that those with clinical obesity have the highest priority for treatments, including weight-loss injections. That said, if you have preclinical obesity I would strongly advise you to consider taking steps to reduce your weight to protect your future health. This might include injections, although depending on your BMI you might need to obtain these via a private prescription, as we will discuss in Chapter 5.

The fact that a group of experts from around the world had to come together to redefine obesity is a sad reflection that as a population we have all got much heavier over the past forty years. In 2022 it was estimated that over 29% of adults in England were obese and a further 35% overweight, which means nearly two-thirds of all adults were either overweight or obese. Read that again – two-thirds of the country's adults are either overweight or obese! Middle-aged adults (between 45 and 64) are the worst affected, with up 40% living with obesity. There are also regional variations, with the highest rate of obesity in the north-west of England (around 35%) and the lowest in London (24%).[6]

Forty years previously, in 1980 obesity only affected around 7% of the population. By 1993, when national records started, this had doubled to around 14%, and by 2003 to 24%. So, in a little over twenty years, obesity rates have more than tripled. Thankfully, the increase has slowed down over the past twenty years, but there is no sign of it tailing off, let alone reversing.

In addition to the impact on adults, in the early 2000s childhood obesity also became a significant concern, affecting about 10% of children under the age of ten. By 2022 over 25% of ten-year-olds were obese and, quite staggeringly, 10% of five-year-olds.[7]

---

[6] Health Survey for England, 2022. https://digital.nhs.uk/data-and-information/publications/statistical/health-survey-for-england/2022-part-2

[7] National Child Measurement Programme. https://digital.nhs.uk/data-and-information/publications/statistical/national-child-measurement-programme/2022-23-school-year

Dr David Cavan

Changing environments change our lifestyles

All the above begs the obvious question: what has changed in our lives over the past few decades to account for such a massive increase in obesity? To help answer this, have a think about what your life is like today compared with when you were a child. What has changed about how we live our lives, how we get about, how we communicate with each other and how we work, play and shop? Well, the first smartphone appeared in 2007, less than twenty years ago. Even if you are only in your thirties, you will be able to remember a time before social media, online shopping and online banking. If you are in your sixties, you will remember a time before fast-food restaurants and coffee shops had appeared on every high street, before freezers and microwaves in the home. You will also remember when most families had one car – if they had one at all – and when many more jobs involved manual and physical work. If you are in your eighties, you will remember food rationing after the war.

The net effect of all these technological advances is that over time our physical activity levels have reduced; we now spend many more hours sitting down than any previous generation in history. Take shopping – before Amazon and other online shopping sites were invented, making any sort of purchase required you to travel to a high street or shopping centre and walk through several shops until you found what you were looking for. Amazon did not exist until 1996, and arrived in the UK in 1998 as a bookseller. Online banking started in the UK in 1997: until then, many of the transactions that we now do routinely via our phone required us to visit our bank. In 1997 only 7% of UK households (and 21% of US households) had access to the internet. The internet has had a greater effect on our lifestyle than any other innovation since the advent of the motor car.

Although cars have been around since the early 1900s, they were the preserve of the rich until much more recently. In 1970, there were under 10 million cars in the UK; by 2020 there were well over 30 million. In that period, the population grew by just over 20%. So, while in the 1970s many families had no car, multiple-car households today are now common.

The other major change to our lives has been to our diet. Imagine for a moment a household that has neither a freezer nor a microwave. What would that mean in terms of the types of food you could eat? It would mean no ice cream or frozen ready meals. No microwave ready meals. In this home, meals were much more likely to be prepared from fresh ingredients each day. And what's the most amazing thing? Until the 1970s, this was reality. Additionally, in the 1970s fast food was a strange American phenomenon rarely found in Europe. I remember visiting the first branch of McDonald's to open in the UK in the late 1970s. The friend I was with was indignant at the absence of knives and forks. 'It won't last long,' he said. The rest, as they say, is history.

When I was young, a can of fizzy drink was a special treat to be enjoyed very occasionally. The same was true for a packet of crisps. Nowadays, many shops in the UK sell a 'meal deal' that typically includes a large bottle of fizzy drink, a sandwich and a packet of crisps. They are bundled together at a good price to entice you to spend a bit extra, and to buy something you probably wouldn't have bought otherwise. The result? That what a couple of generations ago was an occasional special treat, is now part of many people's everyday diet. I recently had a wake-up experience when travelling on a train, sitting behind a group of youngsters from Italy. They were practising their English and I was wryly amused, and at the same time rather ashamed, to hear them make fun of the famous 'meal deal' – highly processed food items that to an Italian would seem quite bizarre – yet it has become, for many people in the UK, the new normal.

Finally, our physical environment can aggravate the effect of other changes to our lifestyle, especially for people who live in a 'food desert'. This is a term to describe areas, often in disadvantaged, low-income neighbourhoods, where there are simply no shops selling healthy foods. I am lucky enough to live in a small town which has one main shopping street along which are a number of outlets selling good-quality fresh foods, including a butcher, two bakers, a delicatessen and a small supermarket (selling meal deals). A few miles down the road are some small villages that either have no shops or one 'convenience store', which is great if you want to buy tobacco, alcohol, sweets or processed foods, but not so great if you want fresh produce. The villages are not served by any bus service, so the only options are to eat what is available at the local shop or drive to the nearest town, where you can buy fresh food. There is the option of ordering online, but that usually comes with a delivery charge that might be unaffordable if money is tight. If you live in an inner-city housing estate with no access to a car, then you have to rely on your local food environment – the food that is available at the nearest shop.

Paradoxically, while fresh food is often hard to find in such places, fast-food outlets are often very common, offering a range of highly processed, unhealthy, albeit relatively inexpensive and accessible foods. It is not surprising that rates of obesity tend to be higher among less advantaged groups, whose food environments are unhealthy and who have limited access to healthy foods.

I saw a very nice example of this when I was visiting a colleague in Nairobi, Kenya. One morning I was sitting at a breakfast table on the terrace of our hotel, enjoying the African sun. On each table was a dish with small packets of sugar for tea or coffee. I watched as a small bird landed on the next table, scooped up a packet of sugar and took off with it. It landed on a wire fence a couple of metres away, pecked open the packet and started to eat the sugar. One of its friends came to perch alongside and they proceeded to share the sugar. Now, I am sure that birds did not evolve to live off highly refined sugar. But this bird was living in an environment where it had become readily available, and it had no need to go foraging.

Our environment isn't finished with us yet – it can also impact on activity levels. 'Walkability' is a term used to describe how easy it is to walk in a particular environment, typically a town or city. This is less of an issue in the UK, but in the USA, many cities are built with cars in mind, not pedestrians. Many main roads were built without any pavement for people to walk safely along. Walkability can also be affected how safe residents think an area is. The provision of cycle lanes also makes a big difference. I am a keen, albeit fair-weather, cyclist, and when I lived in Belgium it was apparent that just about every road had a proper, dedicated cycle path, *for cyclists only*, not a narrow strip of the main road where cyclists have to navigate around parked cars, and not a cycle path that disappears suddenly or decants you either onto the pavement or in the road because the road itself has narrowed. The huge increase in cycling in London over the past twenty years has been a great success, and has benefited many people. However, the narrow roads and lack of cycle lanes has also led to injury and death through collisions with cars and lorries. If people feel safe, they are more likely to cycle; if not, they will use their car.

I have highlighted these examples to illustrate how our lifestyles have changed over the past few decades. This has happened largely because of changes to our environment – food, technological and physical. And, alongside these changes in lifestyle we have witnessed significant adverse changes in our health, with epidemiologically huge increases in obesity across all ages.

Ultra-processed foods

One of the biggest factors in our existing food environment linked to the rise in rates of obesity is how a very high percentage of our diet consists of ultra-processed foods. It may not come as too much of a surprise to learn that the UK is the European champion consumer of ultra-processed foods, which make up over 50% of all the food we eat.[8] This compares with just 14% in Italy (no wonder the students on the train were so shocked by meal deals!).

Historically, foods were processed using salt, drying, fermenting or smoking to preserve them. Such minimally processed foods include cured meats, fish, cheese and other dairy products. Of course, the food industry has developed processing techniques to develop products that bear very little relation to any natural food. Take the crisp-like snack Pringles, for example. They contain starch that originally came from potatoes, but the final product barely resembles a potato. Such snacks and other processed foods are not processed simply to make them last longer; they are formulated very carefully to make us experience all sorts of pleasurable sensations as we eat them – and crucially, to make us want to eat more. Not surprisingly, in recent years we have seen the emergence of the concept of food addiction – or more accurately, addiction to ultra-processed foods.

Many people will relate to the idea of having favourite foods: foods they like so much they can't get enough of them. We often use the term 'moreish' to describe them, as in 'these biscuits are so moreish', which means 'I enjoy these biscuits

---

8 Rauber F, et al. 'Ultra-processed foods and excessive free sugar intake in the UK: A nationally representative cross-sectional study.' *BMJ Open*, 2019, 9: e027546. doi:10.1136/bmjopen-2018-027546

so much I want more'. For some it is cheese, for some it is bread, and for others chocolate or biscuits or ice cream. Very rarely do I hear people describe broccoli or spinach as moreish. If we are able to control our intake of our favourite foods, then our liking for them would not be a problem. However, it is increasingly clear that some people cannot control how much they eat, and they will even behave as if they are addicted to certain foods, in much the same way as people can become addicted to alcohol or drugs.

I can certainly relate to this. I find ice cream, especially good-quality ice cream, extremely moreish. So much so, if there is a tub of ice cream in the freezer, I find it very difficult not to eat it. And I have been known to eat a very large amount in one go. Eating ice cream gives me an immediate pleasurable sensation, beyond the taste itself, that drives me to keep on eating it. Consequently, ice cream is one type of food that I try to avoid having in the house, because I know I *will* eat it. Once upon a time I had a similar relationship with milk chocolate, but since I switched to 70% or higher dark chocolate I find milk chocolate unpleasantly sweet. Yet, notwithstanding the over-sweetness that is no longer to my taste, if I do eat milk chocolate it still has a moreish attraction that will have me going back for more. Sometimes you can't rationalise these things away. The other food that has that effect on me is bread. Not the highly processed white bread you find in supermarkets, but freshly baked sourdough, especially the kind with seeds embedded in its crust.

Some people report that, not only do they lack control when eating certain foods, but if they don't have them at home, they will make a trip to buy some, just like a smoker who has run out of cigarettes will walk through the rain to the corner shop to buy more. Why is this?

A lot of research has investigated the effects of different foods on the brain, and it appears that some foods have addictive effects, just like alcohol and drugs do. Sugar especially stimulates the pleasure centres of the brain and leads to the secretion of dopamine, which has a great feel-good effect. These effects are particularly marked with fructose, the sugar found in fruit. In addition, fructose counteracts the effect of leptin, the hormone we produce when we are full, to tell us to stop eating. Fructose also increases the accumulation of fat in the liver: a key step in the development of insulin resistance, Type 2 diabetes and other health problems that can be associated with obesity. The sugar that is added to foods is usually sucrose (table sugar), which is made up of 50% fructose and 50% glucose. Many processed foods and drinks have high-fructose corn syrup (HFCS) instead, which can be as much as 90% fructose. So you can see how any food with added sugar will encourage you to eat more of it *and* could increase your risk of accumulating excess liver fat.

Sugar has similar properties to alcohol (making you want more and increasing fat in the liver), and I believe there is a valid argument to treat sugar in the same way we legislate around alcohol consumption: by restricting its availability to avoid the harm that arises to those who consume it to excess.

The addictive effects of sugar help to explain my relationship with ice cream and chocolate. Remember that I also have trouble controlling the amount of bread I eat? Bread has very little, if any, sugar in it. But it is high in starch, which is sugar molecules joined together. When these separate, they become glucose. This process begins as we chew bread (and other starchy foods), thanks to the enzyme amylase in our saliva. Some people can taste the sweetness within a few seconds of chewing. So, it is easy to see that addiction to bread, for example, is a variation on sugar addiction. The term 'carb addiction' is also sometimes used to include addiction to starchy foods.

There is evidence that fat has similar, but less marked, effects. However, the combination of sugar and fat has been found to be particularly effective at stimulating addictive overeating. Where do we find that combination? Yes, you've probably guessed it – in all the most addictive foods, including cakes, biscuits and ice cream. And pizza. Some companies add HFCS to pizza crust to give it that golden-brown colour – and a cynic might say they also know that adding sugar increases the addictiveness of pizza, making us want to buy a super-size that we really don't need. The food industry exploits the addictiveness of certain ingredients and has developed a real expertise in adjusting the ingredients in their products, precisely to make us want to eat more. Then they market those products with advertising that is designed to trigger certain feelings – such as seeking happiness – that make us want to buy the product.

If you recognise that you might be addicted to certain foods, it can be difficult to get help as this is not classified as an eating disorder, and it's not generally covered by addiction services. Knowing that certain foods *are* unhealthy is often not enough to make you change what you eat. The cravings are too strong. And as with any addiction, moderation or cutting down is not the answer. It will not work over the longer term. Start by recognising that you need help to cut out such foods altogether. This is one situation where weight-loss injections can really help, as they appear to reduce food cravings, as we will discuss in Chapter 6.

Thankfully, the dangers of ultra-processed foods are now being recognised. Many countries have now introduced different variations of a sugar tax, usually on sugar-sweetened drinks. This was first introduced in Mexico in 2014, and within a short time it had led to a decrease in the consumption of sugary drinks and an increase in the consumption of plain water. The UK followed suit in 2018, but the government gave the drinks industry two years' notice so they had time to reformulate their products to reduce their sugar content and avoid the tax. As a result, the overall consumption of sugar by adults reduced by 10.9 grams every day.[9] Despite the 'sugar tax', many shops sell sugary (full-fat) versions of drinks at the same price as the diet versions, so there is no financial incentive for the purchaser to choose the sugar-free option.

Why do we become obese?

So far, this chapter has discussed what obesity is and how changes to our lifestyles over recent years have led to big increases in obesity rates in the UK and in many other countries across the globe. So let's take a closer look at what happens in our bodies to make us gain weight.

To begin with, humans possess a very efficient energy storage system known as fat. Think of squirrels, which have an abundance of food – such as acorns – each autumn. There are so

---

[9] Rogers NT, et al. 'Estimated changes in free sugar consumption one year after the UK soft drinks industry levy came into force: Controlled interrupted time series analysis of the National Diet and Nutrition Survey (2011–2019).' *J. Epidemiol. Community Health*, 2024, 78: 578–84.

many that the squirrels can eat as many as they like and still have plenty left over, many of which they bury so that when winter comes and food grows scarcer, they can dig them up to eat. Grizzly bears use a different storage method. These huge animals can weigh up to 360 kilograms (800 pounds). They hibernate over winter, but before hibernation they gorge on foods that are plentiful in autumn, particularly fruits, berries, nuts and seeds. This is called hyperphagia (which means overeating), and during this time they can gain 140 kg (300 pounds). This extra weight that comes from the excess calories is stored as fat, and the bear's metabolism slowly uses this fat during its hibernation.

Unlike grizzly bears, we do not hibernate, but we do have a similar evolutionary mechanism that enables us to store excess calories as fat, either under the skin (subcutaneous fat) or in and around our organs, such as the liver (visceral fat). This fat is stored when food is plentiful, and called upon by our bodies when food is unavailable. It was life-saving for our hunter-gatherer ancestors, who did not have the convenience of farmed (and therefore storable) foods or the modern-day ability to acquire calorie-dense foodstuffs at any time of the day or night. They would often have gone for days on end with relatively little to eat. And when they did eat, the energy (calories) in the food was used to immediately fuel the body while the excess was stored as fat that could then be broken down to provide energy later, in times of food scarcity. The trouble is that nowadays in Western societies food (including ultra-processed foods) is always available, so many of us live in a state of constant feast and *no* famine. Our bodies, of course, still use the biological equivalent of the software they have used since the arrival of modern humans 250,000 years ago – very efficiently preserving excess calories as fat for when the lean times come. Except today the lean times don't come, of course, and so, slowly but surely, our body weight increases and people become obese.

While eating more than you need is the trigger that starts the obesity disease process, other factors then come into play to accelerate the process. This is because of the effect of excess weight (or more specifically fat) on our hormones. Hormones are substances produced in one part of the body that enter the bloodstream and influence the cells in different parts of the body. One of the most well-known hormones is insulin, which regulates blood glucose levels. Glucose is a type of sugar that is used for energy by nearly all cells in the body, and it is essential that all parts of the body have a steady supply of glucose. This glucose is obtained from the food we eat: all carbohydrates (sugars and starches) that we eat are broken down into glucose, which is then absorbed from the gut into the bloodstream so it can be carried to the tissues and used as energy. Any spare glucose is taken up into the muscles and liver, where it is stored in the form of glycogen. Glycogen in the muscles is then available for later use if the muscles need extra energy (for example, during intensive exercise). Once our glycogen stores are full, any excess glucose is converted to fat and stored in the liver.

While glucose only enters the body when we eat or drink, the body's cells require a constant supply of glucose to function properly. The liver provides this service by releasing some of its stored glucose into the bloodstream, ensuring that just the right amount of glucose is available during periods when we are not eating (overnight, for example). In a person without diabetes, the amount of glucose in the bloodstream is kept at around 4–6 mmol per litre (70–100 mg/dl).

The level of glucose in the bloodstream is controlled by insulin, which is produced by the pancreas, an organ that sits just below the rib cage, behind the stomach. Like many of the body's organs, the pancreas does a lot of things. However, it has two main functions: one is to produce enzymes that are released directly into the small intestine to break down food so it can be absorbed into the bloodstream. These enzymes include amylase, which breaks down starch into glucose; lipase, which breaks down fat; and protease, which breaks down proteins.

The other main function of the pancreas is to produce hormones. Insulin is one of the hormones produced by the pancreas, and its job is to regulate the amount of glucose in the bloodstream, ensuring that cells always get the right amount of glucose. It does this in several ways:

1. When we eat a meal, the carbohydrate in the meal is converted into glucose in the gut and passes through the gut wall into the bloodstream. The body detects that the glucose level in the blood is rising, and this leads to the pancreas producing additional insulin.
2. This insulin acts on individual cells to allow glucose to enter them. Insulin molecules attach to a receptor on the cell membrane that opens to allow glucose to enter. Insulin is often likened to a 'key' that opens the cell's 'door', allowing glucose to enter the cell.
3. Insulin also stops the liver and muscles from releasing stored glucose into the blood; this allows spare glucose to be added to the glycogen stores.

When we are not eating, the pancreas continually produces a small amount of insulin that controls the release of glucose from the liver. In the liver, insulin acts like a tap that turns off the release of glucose from the organ. If glucose levels in the blood drop too low, then less insulin will be produced (opening the tap), allowing more glucose to be released from the liver. On the other hand, if glucose levels rise then more insulin is produced, closing the tap and slowing down the release of glucose from the liver.

The actions of insulin are extremely well controlled and finely tuned to ensure that the amount of glucose in the blood remains at the optimum level for the body's systems to function. In someone who is overweight, insulin does not work so efficiently, and this accelerates the obesity disease process. Remember that one of the important roles of insulin is to transport glucose into the body's cells. When someone has taken in more energy than they need via their food and drink, the body's cells are so full of glucose that when insulin opens the cell doors, there is no room for the glucose to enter. This means that the glucose stays in the blood, and if the person continues to eat, the level of glucose in the blood will increase. When this happens, the pancreas produces more insulin to try to push the glucose into the cells. But since the cells are already full, the excess glucose is taken up into the liver instead, where it is stored as glycogen. The liver can only store a certain amount of glycogen, and when the glycogen storage area is full, the excess glucose is converted into fat and stored in the liver. Unlike glycogen, it appears that the liver can store almost unlimited amounts of fat – a bit of a design flaw, because when the liver becomes overrun by fat, it begins to leak glucose from the glycogen storage area. It's as if the fat-containing stores bulge out into the glycogen store, forcing the glucose stored there to leak out of the liver and back into the bloodstream. As we have learned, in the liver insulin is a bit like a tap: it regulates the flow of glucose from the glycogen store in the liver into the bloodstream in a very controlled way. Now imagine the increased pressure in those stores because they are being squeezed by the fat all around them. The tap cannot contain the pressure, and the glucose leaks out and into the blood.

So, despite higher insulin levels in the blood, the glucose level in the blood increases still further. This leads to a vicious cycle with the pancreas producing more insulin, leading to more fat being stored in the liver. A high insulin level is known as hyperinsulinaemia (literally high blood insulin), and the leaking insulin tap in the liver is indicative of insulin resistance: that is, the body no longer responds normally to the action of insulin.

This is particularly relevant when discussing obesity, as most people who are obese show signs of hyperinsulinaemia and insulin resistance, and these lead to several of the health problems associated with clinical obesity. Those who do not develop insulin resistance or hyperinsulinaemia are more likely to store fat under the skin (subcutaneous fat) rather than in the liver (visceral fat). They may also have genetic traits or healthier lifestyles that protect them against hyperinsulinemia, and will therefore be more likely to have preclinical obesity without the other associated health problems.

One of the effects of hyperinsulinaemia is to increase hunger, which is why many overweight people struggle to restrict their eating. This is exacerbated by eating ultra-processed foods, as these usually don't make you feel full or satisfy the appetite. They are often also high in sugar and other refined carbohydrates. As these are the foods that most increase insulin levels, you can see why they accelerate the vicious cycle of the obesity disease process.

Another important hormone that is affected in obesity is leptin. Leptin is released by fat cells in the body to regulate hunger and satiety. The more body fat a person has, the more leptin their body produces. This leptin then acts on the hypothalamus in the brain to promote satiety (feeling full) and reduce appetite. A person with low body fat produces less leptin: this promotes feelings of hunger, to encourage the person to eat more to build up their fat stores.

Just as a person with obesity develops insulin resistance, they can also develop leptin resistance. It is as if the brain gets used to chronically high levels of leptin and so stops responding to it, exacerbating the increased hunger that also results from high insulin levels. For leptin to have an effect on the hypothalamus, it must cross the blood–brain barrier – specialised cells that regulate what enters the brain tissue from the bloodstream. There is some evidence that, in obesity, increased inflammation can impair the transport of leptin into the brain, which means that although leptin levels in the blood are high, the brain does not receive the signal to stop eating.

So we can see that, apart from the effect of eating excess calories, which increases body fat, obesity is accelerated by insulin resistance and leptin resistance, compounded by the wide availability of high-calorie, low-satiety, ultra-processed foods. Weight-loss injections help by reducing leptin and insulin resistance.

Other health problems associated with obesity

Metabolic disorders

Insulin resistance is an example of a metabolic disorder. This means that the body's chemical reactions for breaking down food into energy do not function properly. As explained in the previous section, in many people obesity is associated with high insulin levels and insulin resistance. For a while the insulin that the body can produce is sufficient to keep glucose levels normal. As the disease process progresses, however, this is no longer the case and glucose levels rise. This leads to prediabetes if the glucose is slightly raised, and then to Type 2 diabetes. These conditions are diagnosed on the basis of blood tests, either to measure the level of glucose when fasting, or the glycosylated haemoglobin level (abbreviated as HbA1c), which gives an overview of glucose levels over the past six to eight weeks. Prediabetes is diagnosed if the fasting glucose is above 5.5 mmol/l (or 100 mg/dl) and Type 2 diabetes if the level is above 7.0 mmol/l (125 mg/dl). Similarly, an HbA1c above 42 mmol/mol (6.0%) indicates prediabetes, and a level above 48 mmol/mol (6.5%) is diagnostic of Type 2 diabetes. Rates of prediabetes and Type 2 diabetes have increased significantly across the globe in recent years. The good news is that we now know that these conditions can be reversed and put into remission. In people with obesity, it is estimated that losing about 15 kg in weight (33 pounds) can lead to remission of Type 2 diabetes. Further information on reversing these conditions can be found in my book, *How to Reverse Type 2 Diabetes and Prediabetes*.[10]

Insulin resistance is also responsible for several other conditions associated with obesity, as part of what is termed the metabolic syndrome. These include high blood pressure, abnormal cholesterol levels (specifically low high-density lipoprotein (HDL) cholesterol and raised triglycerides) and an increased risk of heart disease. Obesity is also responsible for increasing fat stores in the liver, leading to abnormalities in liver enzymes. This condition used to be called fatty liver

---

[10] Cavan, D. (2024) *How to Reverse Type 2 Diabetes and Prediabetes*. London: Atlantic Books.

and is now known as metabolic dysfunction-associated steatotic liver disease (MASLD). This can progress to metabolic dysfunction-associated steatohepatitis (or MASH), where the excess fat in the liver leads to inflammatory changes in the liver. This can lead to scarring or fibrosis that affects the ability of the liver to function, and can eventually progress to cirrhosis. Cirrhosis indicates that much of the liver has been scarred, and can lead to liver failure or liver cancer. Fortunately, these most advanced stages are quite uncommon, although the milder stages are increasingly common. As with Type 2 diabetes, lifestyle changes leading to weight loss can reduce the fat in the liver, repairing the damage and restoring it to health.

Cardiovascular diseases

In addition to causing high blood pressure, the high insulin levels and insulin resistance associated with clinical obesity can set off several changes that can lead to atherosclerosis (narrowing of the arteries), which reduces the blood flow through them. This can lead to damage to the organs the arteries supply, leading to an increased risk of heart attack or stroke. High insulin levels also increase water retention in the circulation, increasing blood pressure. These changes also increase the risk of chronic kidney disease.

Respiratory issues

Increased fat in the neck can affect breathing, particularly during sleep, and can cause obstructive sleep apnoea. This is characterised by snoring and periods when breathing stops (apnoea). Often the person does not wake up fully when this happens, but their sleep is sufficiently disturbed to cause excessive tiredness and sleepiness during the day, which can have a significant impact on their quality of life.

Excess fat in the rib cage and abdomen can reduce the ability of the lungs to expand fully when breathing, causing shortness of breath.

Hormonal disorders

In addition to the effect on insulin and leptin levels, obesity can affect other hormones, particularly the sex hormones. Polycystic ovary syndrome (PCOS) is a common condition in women, and largely results from an imbalance of sex hormones, which is caused by insulin resistance. This can lead to weight gain and an excess of testosterone, which can lead to increased body hair and male-pattern scalp baldness. It also leads to infrequent or absent periods and infertility. Weight reduction and medication that reduces insulin resistance can be very effective in reversing these trends and restoring fertility. In men, testosterone is converted to oestrogen in fat, and this process is enhanced in people with obesity. Obesity can also affect levels of the hormones secreted by the pituitary gland that regulate the level of testosterone and sperm production. As well as affecting libido and fertility, in men low testosterone is associated with weight gain, setting up an additional vicious cycle. It is also associated with low mood, and this can make it more difficult for an individual to lose weight.

Digestive problems

Excess fat in the abdomen can put pressure on the stomach, effectively squeezing the acid in the stomach into the oesophagus, irritating its lining, which causes gastroesophageal reflux disease (GERD). High levels of cholesterol in the bile of people with obesity increases the risk of gallstones.

Joint and musculoskeletal issues

Excess weight puts pressure on joints and damages cartilage, to cause osteoarthritis. This causes pain and restriction of movement, especially in the hips, knees and spine.

Mental health and neurological effects

High insulin levels in obesity can affect how the chemical connectors between brain cells (neurotransmitters) work, leading to reduced cognitive function (commonly described as brain fog) and mood disorders. Insulin resistance also increases the risk of depression and, in the longer term, dementia.

Cancer risk

Many types of cancer have become more common as obesity rates have increased. Obesity is associated with an increased risk of breast cancer, womb (uterus) cancer, bowel cancer, pancreatic cancer and liver cancer.

Obesity is associated with many other problems, such as urinary incontinence, due to weakened pelvic floor muscles and chronic inflammation, as fat cells release cytokines that stimulate inflammation.

This long and rather depressing list demonstrates how clinical obesity affects many different aspects of health. This is why it's so important to lose weight permanently to reverse these problems, where possible, and to prevent them causing further ill health. Losing weight will require significant lifestyle changes.

A Guide to Weight Loss Injections

Chapter 3 describes the healthy eating changes that I recommend you make before you start taking weight-loss injections.

Chapter 3
Eating for success on weight-loss injections

In Chapter 2 we learned that the main reason that so many people have become obese in recent years is because our lifestyles have changed so dramatically, and we are eating too much. The key to successful weight loss is to make permanent changes to your lifestyle. These changes are *essential* to a successful and long-lasting outcome, even if you are going to embark on weight-loss injections. In the USA these treatments are licensed for long-term treatment, but in the UK the National Health Service (NHS) will only provide Wegovy for up to two years. I agree with this approach, as we do not yet know how safe these treatments are when taken for multiple years. This means that after two years you will need to come off the injections – and unless you have trained yourself to live and eat in a different way, it is likely that the pounds will pile back on again. This has been widely reported in newspapers, magazines and on social media by people who have already experienced precisely that. So, before we even start to discuss using weight-loss injections to lose weight, this chapter will describe the changes to your diet and lifestyle that I believe are essential for successful long-term weight loss. These changes are also designed to maximise the effectiveness of weight-loss injections and reduce their side effects, when you do take them.

Diet changes

Many overweight people struggle to lose weight for years or even decades, despite trying all manner of diets. I believe that the key to successful long-term weight loss is to move away from thinking about a diet as such. Instead, you should think about a **permanent change in eating habits**. So, these changes must be sustainable in the long term. As we all have different tastes and preferences, and different relationships with food, I do not provide a prescriptive diet that you must follow. Rather, I suggest changes that in my experience are most likely to help promote weight loss, and leave it to you to decide which changes to make, in which order, so they work best for you and your circumstances.

For countless years the official advice on diet in the UK (and in many other countries) has been to follow a low-fat, high-fibre diet with around a third of each meal based on starchy carbohydrates. This forms the basis of the Eatwell Guide. However, as many people have discovered, this approach does not help weight loss. Let me explain why I think the advice found in the Eatwell Guide (Figure 3.1) is inappropriate for a person trying to lose weight.

Figure 3.1. The Eatwell Guide: official dietary advice from the UK government.

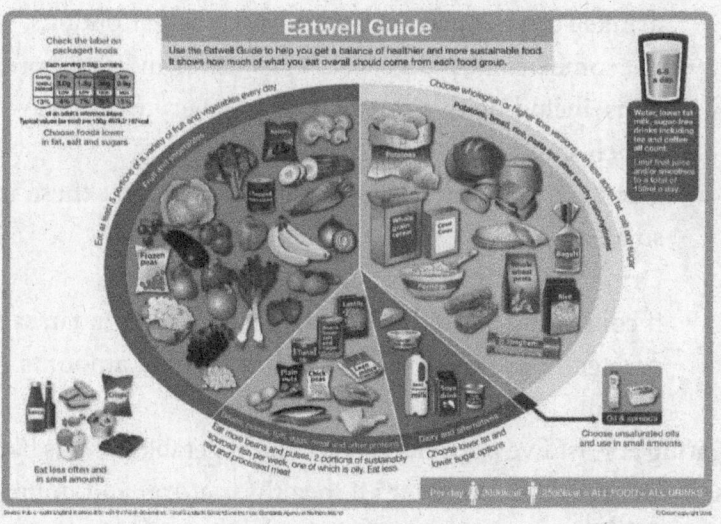

Source: Crown copyright. OHID in association with the Welsh government, Food Standards Scotland and the Food Standards Agency in Northern Ireland.

Its main recommendations are:[11]

- Eat at least five portions of a variety of fruit and vegetables every day.
- Base meals on potatoes, bread, rice, pasta or other starchy carbohydrates, choosing wholegrain versions where possible.
- Have some dairy or dairy alternatives (such as soya drinks), choosing lower fat and lower sugar options.
- Eat some beans, pulses, fish, eggs, meat and other proteins (including two portions of fish every week, one of which should be oily).
- Choose unsaturated oils and spreads, and eat these in small amounts.
- Drink six to eight cups/glasses of fluid a day.
- If consuming foods and drinks that are high in fat, salt or sugar, have these less often and in small amounts.

Eating at least five portions of fruit and vegetables seems like a good idea: they are, after all, healthy, natural and unprocessed foods. However, in Chapter 2 we learned that many people living with obesity have high insulin levels, which drive fat storage and further weight gain. Insulin is secreted

---

[11] The NHS Eatwell Guide. https://www.nhs.uk/live-well/eat-well/how-to-eat-a-balanced-diet/eating-a-balanced-diet

by the pancreas when we eat, and the most insulin is produced when we eat foods that contain carbohydrates – that is, sugars or starches. There is very little carbohydrate in leafy and salad vegetables. Cabbage, courgette, cucumber, tomatoes and cauliflower, for example, all have around 3% or less carbohydrate (excluding fibre, which, strictly speaking, is a carbohydrate, but is not digested so is not counted). Lettuce, spinach, asparagus, olives and avocado contain even less. Root vegetables such as celeriac or carrots are pretty low with 7%, whereas potatoes have about 15%. But what about fruit? Bananas can have as much as 20% carbs and grapes have 16%. And raisins have about 75% carbohydrate! Yet in the Eatwell Guide, these are all lumped together. Why? Because this advice was not designed with its impact on insulin levels in mind. According to the Eatwell Guide, fruit and vegetables are all healthy because they contain fibre and plenty of vitamins and minerals. But a tomato or a few chunks of cucumber will have negligible effect on insulin levels and fat storage, whereas a banana could have a massive impact. A large ripe banana could contain up to 40 grams of carbohydrate, most of which is sugar, yet many people have been recommended to eat this as a healthy snack. I would argue that even for a person with a healthy metabolism, consuming this amount of sugar cannot be construed as being good for you.

Turning to starches, remember these are simply sugar molecules ($C_6H_{10}O_5$) joined together (known as a polymer of glucose). As soon as starch enters your mouth, it begins to break down into its constituent glucose. This glucose can enter the bloodstream very quickly after eating foods such as bread and white rice, leading to a rapid increase in insulin levels. Other foods, such as pasta, will cause a slower rise. Even porridge, which is almost universally believed to be a good thing, is over 60% carbohydrate and will cause a big, sustained rise in glucose and insulin levels.

The NHS advice is to choose wholegrain versions wherever possible. This is because whole grains contain more fibre, and this slows down the rise in blood glucose. Yet wholegrain bread, pasta and cereals contain so much carbohydrate that they still have a big impact in increasing insulin levels.

These two categories of food (fruit/vegetables and starches) cover three-quarters of the plate. Anyone following the Eatwell Guide will therefore have a high intake of starches and, depending on the fruits they choose, sugars. What would this type of diet do to the vicious cycle that is the obesity disease process? Sugars and starches cause blood glucose to rise, prompting the pancreas to release more insulin. High levels of glucose lead to high levels of insulin. High levels of insulin lead to excess energy being stored as fat in the liver. Fat in the liver is a key step in the development of insulin resistance, that leads to the health problems we discussed in

Chapter 2. Basing all meals on starchy carbohydrates will only continue that cycle.

It comes as no surprise to me that rates of obesity have skyrocketed since the 1980s, when dietary guidelines first recommended a low-fat, high-carbohydrate diet. And it doesn't take a genius to work out that changing to a diet that consists of foods that do not increase blood glucose would be a good change to make. Rather than basing all meals on starchy carbohydrates, I firmly believe that the best eating pattern for a person who wants to lose weight is one that **restricts carbohydrates** to a greater or lesser extent, according to personal preference and an individual's goals for their health.

Perhaps because so many people have found the official advice doesn't work, there has been an explosion in interest in alternative diets in recent years. These include plant-based diets, ketogenic (keto) diets (which are very low in carbohydrate and high in fat), low-carbohydrate diets and most recently carnivore diets (which exclude all plant-based foods). I leave it to each reader to decide the approach that best suits them, but what all these approaches have in common is that they are based on restricting carbohydrates.

Since all plant sources of protein (such as beans or lentils) contain carbohydrates, plant-based diets generally involve a higher carbohydrate intake. However, if you reduce or exclude sugars and other refined carbohydrates (such as white bread, pasta and rice) and ultra-processed foods (UPFs), it is perfectly possible to make real health improvements by eating a plant-based diet. Excluding meat can increase the risk of nutritional deficiencies, such as vitamin B12 or iron, so I generally recommend that if you exclude meat from your diet you take any necessary supplements.

Another diet that has gained a lot of attention is the Mediterranean diet. This is a bit of a misnomer as the Mediterranean is surrounded by many different countries and cultures, some of which have diets that traditionally contain a lot of starches, such as rice or bread. A key part of the Mediterranean diet is a high intake of fresh vegetables, healthy fats (as found in oily fish and olive oil), minimally processed dairy produce and fresh, unprocessed meat. Remember that the UK is the processed food champion of Europe and how the Italians I came across mocked the Great British Meal Deal? Guess what? A traditional Mediterranean diet is low in UPFs. The Mediterranean diet has several health benefits and a study published in 2013 demonstrated that eating a Mediterranean diet was associated with a 30% reduction in cardiovascular events (e.g. heart attacks or strokes) compared to eating a low-fat diet.[12]

---

[12] Estruch R, Ros E, Salas-Salvado J, et al. 'Primary prevention of cardiovascular disease with a Mediterranean diet.' *N. Engl. J. Med.*, 2013, 368: 1279–90.

Healthy choices and how to integrate them

Rather than get bogged down in definitions or precise diet plans, my approach is to suggest a simple, step-by-step approach. If you want to lose weight, a priority must be to reduce the insulin in your bloodstream. Not only will this help to reduce fat storage, it will also reduce the feelings of hunger that drive so many people to overeat.

Nearly all foods have some effect on blood insulin levels, but by far the biggest culprits are sugars and starches. Therefore, my first recommendation is to reduce these. Since we don't always know what is in processed foods, my second recommendation is to make sure you know what you are eating – and that means eating fresh, unprocessed foods, as far as possible. So, what does that mean in practice?

1. *Cut out sugars*

This is essential. If you were my new patient, one of my first questions would be: are you willing to try to cut out sugars as much as possible? It doesn't mean never eating any foods containing sugar (frankly, that would be nigh on impossible), but it does mean not including sugary foods as part of your daily diet. Minimising sugars is essential to reduce insulin levels. Apart from the obvious (sugary drinks, sweets, desserts, cakes and biscuits), it also includes many processed foods (such as baked beans and tinned tomato soup). It also includes natural sugars or syrups (such as honey) and fruit that is high in sugar (such as bananas, grapes (unless you can limit yourself to just a few), pineapple and large apples, pears and oranges (small ones are okay, but still not ideal).

If you are alarmed by the idea of never eating sweet treats again, then you could investigate low-sugar alternatives that use artificial sweeteners. Otherwise, save sweet treats for the (very) infrequent special occasion. Allow yourself a small piece of cake to celebrate a birthday, and accept that it will cause your insulin level to rise and your body to store the excess energy as fat, but you are willing to take this risk to share in the celebration.

If you have been told that you can eat anything in moderation, and especially if you have been encouraged to eat a lot of fruit, cutting out sugar could mean a big change to your current eating pattern. However, you don't have to change everything in one go. It's important that you set yourself goals to make changes that are realistic for you, and that you can stick to.

2. *Avoid ultra-processed foods*

Many ultra-processed foods (UPFs) contain high levels of sugars, harmful trans fats (discussed in more detail later in this chapter) and all sorts of other chemicals. I have recently heard UPFs being referred to as 'recreational drugs'. Given the lengths to which the food industry goes to make UPFs as tasty and as moreish as possible, this is a perfectly apt description. I strongly recommend that you try to limit UPFs as much as you can. A good way to start is to buy foods that **do not have an ingredients list** (such as fresh meat and vegetables), or to buy foods that have no more than five ingredients (minimally processed foods such as cooked meat, butter or cheese). Butter has just one ingredient – milk – whereas margarine and other so-called heathy butter alternatives can have eleven or twelve more, including colouring, flavourings, stabilisers and emulsifiers to recreate the buttery taste and texture.

3. *Reduce starches*

Starches are found in white or beige foods, including bread, potatoes, rice, pasta, cereals and any foods that contain flour. Remember what I said earlier? Starch is simply glucose molecules stuck together, and some starchy foods, such as white rice, can push up your blood glucose (and hence insulin) level faster than eating a bowlful of sugar. Here's a trick: close your eyes and visualise your bowl of rice, pasta, breakfast cereal or potatoes as a bowl of sugar: as far as your body is concerned, that is essentially what it is. Your body responds by releasing a lot of insulin to store the excess energy as fat. Refined carbohydrates can also worsen some of the side effects of weight-loss injections, so when you have started taking the injections I recommend that you avoid large portions of starchy foods. This means not eating meals based on pasta, rice, pastry or potato and breakfast cereals. Instead, base your meals on meat or another form of protein and plenty of vegetables, with, at most, a small portion of starchy food as part of the meal. Or experiment with alternatives, such as making 'rice' from grated cauliflower or mixed vegetables to eat with a curry, or having courgette strips or leek ribbons instead of pasta.

While white and beige foods contain the highest amounts of starch, smaller amounts are also found in pulses (peas, beans and lentils) and root vegetables (parsnips and carrots). These are also high in fibre, which helps to reduce their impact on blood glucose and insulin levels.

4. *Prioritise protein*

If you reduce starches in your meals but make no other changes to your diet, then you may find that you go hungry. This is counterproductive. When you are hungry you will end up eating any food you have in the house, and it could well be high in carbohydrate. So, if you are reducing carbohydrates, make sure you fill up with foods that will not increase the level of glucose (and therefore insulin) in your blood. I usually suggest increasing the protein in your meals. Protein is found in meat, fish, eggs, cheese, pulses and nuts. While protein has some effect in increasing blood glucose levels, it is much less than carbohydrates, so there is no insulin surge to make you hungry again a short time later. Meals that contain protein stay in the stomach for longer, so you feel fuller for longer after eating them, and feel less need to snack a couple of hours later. If you do get hungry between meals, try eating a hard-boiled egg or a tinned sardine. They are inexpensive, nutritious, high-protein real foods with next to no carbohydrate, and they are very filling – so much so, it is almost impossible to eat a second one. Now, you can't say the same about biscuits...

Protein is essential to maintain muscle strength. With many weight-loss diets, a good proportion of the weight lost is muscle mass, which risks further health problems due to muscle weakness and frailty in later life. As we will discuss in more detail in Chapter 7, weight-loss injections are associated with loss of muscle mass, so it is a good idea to start prioritising protein before you start taking them.

5. *Don't fear fat*

Low-fat foods were introduced in the 1970s, as it was thought that eating saturated fat increased the risk of heart disease.

This was called the diet–heart hypothesis, and it led to governments in many countries recommending that we should all eat a low-fat diet. The food industry responded by removing fat from many natural foods, such as dairy products, and adding sugar to make up for their lack of taste – essentially creating a huge array of processed foods. More recent studies have questioned the link between fat and heart disease. In 2017, a large study[13] looked at the diets of over 130,000 people in 18 countries and found that there was **no association between fat intake and cardiovascular disease**. In fact, a higher fat intake was associated with a reduced risk of death, whereas those who had a higher carbohydrate intake were more likely to die.

Many people believe that fat is bad. I have had to repeat endlessly to my patients that it is not just okay to eat fat, but it is better than eating carbohydrates. There are many types of fat – monounsaturated, polyunsaturated (omega 3 and omega 6), saturated and trans fats. While some are certainly bad, most are now recognised to be very good for us.

Monounsaturated fat is found in olives, seeds and various types of nuts. Nuts have a low carbohydrate content, and are quite high in mainly healthy fats, meaning they can satisfy

---

[13] Dehghan M, et al. 'Associations of fats and carbohydrate intake with cardiovascular disease and mortality in 18 countries from five continents (PURE): A prospective cohort study.' *Lancet*, 2017, 390(10107): 2050–62.

the appetite: a handful of nuts is a good snack. What is also overlooked, or at least understated, is that about half of the fat in meat (including red meat) is also monounsaturated. I therefore regard all types of unprocessed meats as nutritious and healthy.

Polyunsaturated fat comes in two types. One is omega 3, which is healthy fat and may help lower the risk of heart disease, depression, dementia and arthritis. Your body can't make it, so you must eat foods that contain it. It is found in oily fish, and ideally should be eaten two to three times a week. Nuts (especially walnuts) and linseed (flaxseed) are also a good source of omega 3. The other type of polyunsaturated fat is omega 6, which is less beneficial. It is found in vegetable oils and spreads containing corn oil or sunflower oil. Eating too many foods containing omega 6 fats can increase inflammation in the body.

Saturated fat is found in dairy products, meat and coconut (and, in small amounts, in avocado). Since 2015, research has shown that saturated fat is not the enemy we once thought it was, and it is not associated with an increased risk of heart disease.[14] It also increases healthy HDL cholesterol levels. In

---

14 de Souza RJ, Mente A, Maroleanu A, et al. 'Intake of saturated and trans unsaturated fatty acids and risk of all cause mortality, cardiovascular disease, and Type 2 diabetes: Systematic review and meta-analysis of observational studies.' *BMJ*, 2015, 351: h3978.

natural foods such as unprocessed meat, it can be considered a healthy fat.

Trans fats (also known as hydrogenated fats) are the real baddies. Although they occur in small quantities in some natural foods, such as meat and dairy products, human-made versions are found in many processed foods. Trans fats are created through the partial hydrogenation of vegetable oils, where hydrogen is added to liquid oils to make them more solid and shelf-stable. They have been shown to increase inflammation and the risk of heart disease. Lots of food manufacturers are reducing their use of trans fats, but they can still be found in many baked products, such as cakes and biscuits, margarines, and in foods fried in vegetable oils.

Adding healthy fats to your diet can help to make meals more filling. Naturally occurring fats as found in oily fish, nuts, avocado and olives are considered healthy. Adding some of these can make a salad into a delicious, filling meal. Fat also has virtually no effect on blood glucose or insulin levels.

Okay ... so what about cheese? There is now evidence from several studies[15] that dairy products are not harmful to our health, and some, such as yoghurt and cheese, may actually

---

15 Forouhi NG, Krauss RM, Taubes G, Willett W. 'Dietary fat and cardiometabolic health: Evidence, controversies, and consensus for guidance.' *BMJ*, 2018, 361: k2139.

be associated with a lower risk of heart disease. You might want to read that sentence again, as it likely flies in the face of everything you have previously heard. So, yes, you can eat cheese. I have lost count of the number of people who are shocked when I say 'Why not eat some cheese?' They feel liberated after many years of being told not to eat it, or that they should only be eating low-fat varieties. I would much rather my patients have a small piece of cheese as a snack than a sweet biscuit. Of course, if you eat a lot of cheese, or other dairy products, then you will gain weight. Since cheese (like nuts) contains small amounts of carbohydrate, it can be rather moreish, and if you are not careful you can end up eating quite a lot. But a small piece of cheese, preferably without a cracker, is a delicious and healthy way to round off a meal.

In summary, dairy products, nuts, seeds, oily fish and meat all contain healthy natural fats and you can enjoy them as part of your eating plan.

6. *Don't count calories*

Most weight-loss diets are based on the principle that you take in fewer calories in food and drink, and you use up more calories by physical activity than you have eaten, and therefore lose weight. Many diets encourage you to count the calories in the foods you eat, to ensure you stick to a certain number. In my experience, many people find such diets hard to follow, so they often do not work.

These diets assume that a calorie from fat has the same effect on your body as a calorie from protein or carbohydrate. In my view, this is a huge oversimplification. We have already heard that protein and fat have a much smaller effect on blood glucose levels than carbohydrate; the body will release much more insulin after a small portion of rice that contains 200 calories than after a piece of cheese that also contains 200 calories. Remember, insulin is the fat storage hormone and more fat is likely to be stored after eating 200 calories in rice than in cheese – even though cheese contains more fat. This serves to remind us that **it is important not to confuse fat as a nutrient with fat as a body tissue**. Yes, they have the same name but they are very different.

Insulin also promotes hunger, so you are more likely to want to eat more after eating rice. A few years ago Sam Feltham, Director of the UK's Public Health Collaboration, did a single-person experiment to assess how different types of foods affect weight. He ate 5,800 calories a day for 21 days, each on two different diets. When he ate a low-carb, high-fat diet his weight increased by 1.3 kg, yet when he ate a low-fat, high-carbohydrate diet, his weight increased by 7.1 kg! But the number of calories he ate was the same. He noted that on the low-carbohydrate diet he wasn't hungry and often had to force himself to eat to make up his target calorie count.[16]

This demonstrated how, through the action of insulin, carbohydrates have a bigger impact on hunger and on body weight than other nutrients. And yet most calorie-controlled diets completely ignore the role of insulin.

Furthermore, some foods use up more energy in their digestion than others. Protein requires up to 30% of its calories to digest it, whereas carbohydrate requires about 10%. So, if you have 200 calories as protein – as in a 200 gram (7 ounce) steak, for example, 60 of those calories are burned off in the digestion process, meaning your body only gets to use 140 of them. On the other hand, only 10% of calories are burned off digesting carbohydrate (20 calories in a small portion of rice). These flaws in the low-calorie argument have led many of us to believe that a calorie in rice or sugar is much more harmful than a calorie in steak or cream – or, to put it another way, not all calories are the same in how they affect your weight.

If you significantly reduce your calorie intake, say to 800 calories a day, then you will likely lose weight. But many people

---

16 Feltham S, Westman EC. 'A case study of overfeeding 3 different diets.' *Curr. Opin. Endocrinol. Diabetes Obes.*, 2021, 28(5): 446–52. doi:10.1097/MED.0000000000000668

find that they can also lose a lot of weight simply by reducing the carbohydrates in their diet. Replacing starchy carbs with green vegetables is a great way to start and will reduce your insulin level, which is – as I keep repeating – key to losing weight, because it reverses the vicious cycle of the obesity disease process.

So, I suggest that you don't need to count calories. Reducing carbohydrates will likely also reduce the calories you eat. Having said that, it is important to be aware of which low-carbohydrate foods are high in calories, such as cheese or nuts, and to limit your intake of these if you are finding it difficult to lose weight.

Making a start on your new diet

So, cutting out sugars and avoiding large portions of starches are important first steps in your weight-loss journey. But how you set about doing that is entirely up to you. Some people choose to cut out all starchy foods and eat a very low-carbohydrate, ketogenic diet. Others follow a carnivore diet, eating only meat, eggs and dairy products. Both will lead to an immediate and dramatic reduction in blood glucose and hence insulin levels, but some people can find these diets too restrictive, and the evidence suggests they are unnecessary for many people. Making severe reductions to carbohydrate intake can lead to side effects, such as constipation, muscle cramps and headaches. These usually subside after a few days and can be eased by drinking plenty of fluids.

So, rather than reducing carbohydrates as much as possible, the most important thing is to choose an eating plan that you think you will be able to stick to over the long term. It is perfectly possible to lose weight sustainably while still enjoying small amounts of starch in your diet.

Many people prefer to make gradual changes to their diet. I have developed a step-by-step approach to reducing carbohydrates. This approach addresses the most important changes first. However, it is not the only way. You may feel that Step 4 is the easiest change for you to make – if so, start with Step 4 rather than Step 1. Please note that if you have diabetes that is managed by medication, it is essential that you discuss any changes to your diet with a health professional, as you may need to reduce the dose of some medications to minimise the risk of hypoglycaemia (an abnormally low blood glucose level).

Step 1: Stop drinking sugary drinks

Cutting out added sugars is probably the most important first step – and if you drink sugary drinks, these should be the first thing you should stop consuming. There is plenty of scientific evidence to show that sugar-sweetened beverages are harmful, so I recommend to my patients they cut them out completely. In addition to the obvious examples, such as Coke and other types of fizzy drink, this will also mean cutting out fruit juices and smoothies, despite the health benefits they may claim. We have already discussed that some fruits are not a healthy option if you want to lose weight, but any fruit when turned into a smoothie becomes a very sweet drink, albeit with some fibre in it. In terms of sugar content, smoothies are on a par with Coke. It does not matter that the sugar is 'natural' (it originally came from fruit) – it is still sugar that will have a significant impact on the level of glucose, and therefore insulin, in your bloodstream. This also means cutting out sweetened hot drinks such as hot chocolate, lattes and flavoured cappuccinos, which are widely available in popular coffee shops.

There are not many things that I suggest avoiding completely, but sweet drinks are one of them. I would go as far as to say that I don't think it's possible to lose weight if you continue to drink sugar in this way. If you like sugary drinks, please consider switching to diet versions that use artificial sweeteners. This is a great first step in reducing your sugar intake. Sweeteners can also cause problems, but they are a much better option than sugar.

To minimise liquid sugar intake, the best drinks are water or unsweetened tea (including fruit or herbal teas) or coffee with a dash of milk. To add flavour to a glass of water, try adding a slice of lemon, lime or cucumber.

Step 2: Reduce snacking

The next stage is to cut right down on sugary foods. Many natural foods have small amounts of sugar, so it is not possible to avoid sugar completely. However, you can try to avoid foods with added sugar, such as sweets, biscuits, cakes, ice cream and desserts, as well as sweet fruit. A lot of these foods are snacks rather than main meals so, rather than focusing on a long list of foods that you need to avoid, I encourage you to think of it another way: as **cutting out snacks**.

Snacks were invented by the food industry to maximise their profits by getting us to eat food we don't need, and the food industry throws hundreds of millions of pounds annually at developing and marketing them. As a child, I remember being told not to snack as it would 'spoil my appetite', but now we are encouraged to get through tons of snacks, many of which are ultra-processed and high in sugar. As a relatively new grandad, I have noticed that toddlers cannot go anywhere without an ultra-processed (often marketed as 'organic') snack readily available, and so we are teaching future generations that this is normal. It is not.

Instead, I encourage you to focus on eating enough in your main meals to fill you up, thereby avoiding the need for any food between meals. That means having your mid-morning cup of tea or coffee on its own, without a biscuit, banana or bar of chocolate, or, if you are in a coffee shop, a cake or pastry. Remember, we do not *need* any of these foods: we eat them because we like them, and quite often because it has become a habit. Yes, we might enjoy the taste and the sugar rush that comes with the first few mouthfuls, but then we might feel rather bloated and uncomfortable afterwards. Try having a drink without a snack: you will find that you can still enjoy your drink, and as it fills your stomach it will make you feel full, but without feeling as if you have overdone it.

If you eat biscuits, chocolate or cake between meals, then cutting them out will reduce your sugar intake very significantly. This will reduce your blood glucose level, which in turn will reduce your insulin level. This means you will feel less hungry between meals, with less need to snack. And will mean your glucose and insulin levels will stay down and you will likely lose weight. Win-win!

There will be times when you feel peckish, so it's important to ensure you have some healthy snacks available. Examples include a small piece of cheese, a few strawberries, some vegetable sticks (carrot or cucumber is good), a handful of nuts, a hard-boiled egg or a piece of dark chocolate.

A Guide to Weight Loss Injections

Maybe you do not eat cakes or biscuits, but you enjoy eating fruit – perhaps five or more pieces a day. You may be thinking you are doing the right thing, as all the official advice is to eat fruit. However, some fruit, such as banana, pineapple and mango, is very high in sugar and are best avoided, unless you can restrict yourself to a very small portion. A single grape is low in sugar, and as long as you eat no more than five at a time, this should be fine: however, if stopping at five is difficult, then it's best to avoid grapes. Instead, get your five a day from vegetables rather than fruit. If you want to enjoy fruit, remember this: berries are best, as they are very low in sugar, followed by small apples, plums or tangerines – or any fruit that you can easily fit in the palm of your hand. Dried fruit (such as prunes, raisins and dried apricots), on the other hand, is very high in sugar, so it is best avoided.

If you have a sweet tooth, or you simply enjoy eating sweet treats, you might find it difficult to cut out sugary foods completely. If that is the case, then start by identifying one or two small changes that you think you can make. It could be having one instead of two biscuits or having an apple instead of a pastry. It doesn't matter what the change is, so long as it is one you think you can achieve. Some people feel that they are addicted to certain foods, usually containing sugar or other refined carbohydrates. If you feel like this, your aim should be that eventually you stop them completely, however difficult that might seem at the start.

Step 3: Have less starch for breakfast

Having reduced your sugar intake, the next step I suggest is to reduce the starchy foods in your diet. Remember the mantra – starch is simply sugar molecules joined together and, like sugar, it increases the glucose and insulin levels in the blood. Reducing starchy foods is therefore an essential part of reversing the obesity disease process.

For Step 3, I suggest focusing on breakfast to start with, and there is a very good reason for this. Whenever I ask people what they eat for breakfast, most say they have starch, in the form of cereal and/or toast. However, breakfast is the worst possible time to challenge the body with carbohydrates. At this time the levels of many hormones – such as cortisol and growth hormone – are quite high. I call them the 'wake up' hormones as they prepare the body for the day ahead, and part of the way they work is to counter the effect of insulin. In other words, insulin resistance is worse at breakfast time than at any other time of the day.

For many people, breakfast means having a breakfast cereal. It was my standard breakfast for countless years. But take a look at the ingredients listed on the box and you will see they are all UPFs. Many so-called 'healthy' options, such as muesli, contain dried fruit and are very high in sugar (even when labelled 'no added sugar'), and they are all very high in starch. As far as your body is concerned, you might as well eat a bowlful of sugar. Many people then eat a slice or two of toast after their cereal, each slice being 15–20 grams of carbohydrate. So a breakfast of a bowl of cereal and couple of slices of toast could easily add up to 80 or 90 grams of carbohydrate, in just one meal, at the time of day when your body is least able to deal with it.

The most important advice I can give here is to stop eating breakfast cereals – all of them, including the so-called healthy ones and porridge. Plain (full-fat) Greek yoghurt with some mixed berries is a natural, filling, healthier alternative, with a fraction of the carbohydrate content. If you have time to cook, bacon and eggs or a mushroom omelette will fill you up and boost your protein intake with practically zero carbs!

Step 4: Have a low-carb lunch

Just as breakfast can add up to a huge carb load, so can lunch – or what has become a usual lunch for many of us. The infamous meal deal of a sandwich, packet of crisps and a drink can easily total over 80 grams of carbohydrate. So what are the options to reduce carbs at lunchtime, especially if you are out and about? Some people ask me if a wrap is a better option than a sandwich, and the answer is emphatically no! A wrap can easily contain the same, if not more, carbohydrate than two slices of bread. The same goes for crackers or crispbread. While they are small and thin, they are basically concentrated flour, and therefore very high in carbohydrate.

If you want a low-carbohydrate lunch, you really need to move away from flour-based foods. My advice is to have soup or salad. A salad has very few carbs, and if you choose carefully, many soups are also low-carb, especially when they are homemade.

Homemade soup, particularly vegetable soup, is remarkably easy to make – even if you don't consider yourself to be a great cook – and is usually very tasty. Add ham or cooked chicken or lentils to provide protein. You can make up a large quantity and take it to work in a container to microwave or in an insulated flask. For salads, I generally say: have whatever protein you would have put in your sandwich, but with some lettuce and tomato instead of bread. Add a hard-boiled egg and you have a high-protein (and therefore very filling) low-carb lunch.

Rather than going to the sandwich aisle for lunch, go to the cooked meat or cheese section. Many supermarkets now sell cooked chicken thighs or drumsticks and slices of ham or cheese that can be eaten 'on the go'. Another option, but one that's less easy to eat on the move, is tinned fish. One of my patients once told me that they take a tin of sardines to work for lunch. It might not be as easy to eat as a sandwich, but with a bit of care, you can eat sardines from the tin at your desk. They are packed with protein and healthy fats, with near-zero carbohydrate. They will likely keep you full right into the evening. In the UK at least, they are also very cheap, at around 60p for a 125-gram tin of sardines in olive oil or brine – much cheaper than any shop-bought sandwich or meal deal.

If you can't avoid eating a sandwich for lunch, I suggest eating sandwiches with the most generous fillings, and eat as few as you need to feel full. If you can, leave the crusts. Or if you're at home, try some of the lower-carb breads that are now available, or buy one of the low-carb alternatives to flour – these can be used to make very passable bread.

Step 5: Think 'meat and two veg'

When it comes to main meals, my advice is to think of 'meat and two veg' type meals rather than meals based on potatoes, pasta or rice. Perhaps 'protein and as many veg as you can manage' is a better description. This is designed to include meals for non-meat eaters and to emphasise the importance of prioritising protein. You can pile your plate with as many veg as you like to fill you up. Steve Bennett in his book *Fibre First* describes some very nice experiments where he monitored the effect of different meals on blood glucose levels in volunteers.[17] He then asked them to have the same meal but to eat high-fibre foods first. These could be leafy green vegetables on the dinner plate, or a salad, carrot sticks or nuts as a starter. This led to a much lower impact on blood glucose levels, and showed how fibre keeps food in the stomach for longer and slows down the absorption of glucose from the gut. This will make you feel fuller for longer so you eat less, so this simple change can help you lose weight.

Note that when you are taking Wegovy or Mounjaro, you will not be able to eat so much, so it is important to get the protein in first rather than filling up on vegetables so you don't have the appetite for protein. When taking injections, it is important to have a good protein intake of at least 1.2 g per kg of body weight (or 0.55 g per pound) every day. If you weigh 80 kg (176 pounds), that means at least 90 g of protein per day. In Chapter 8, I suggest 20–40 grams of protein with each meal and give examples of how you can achieve this – including using protein shakes if your appetite for solid food is reduced. So, any type of meat, poultry, fish, seafood, pulses, nuts, seeds, cheese or eggs prepared in any way you choose.

---

17 Bennett, S (2024), *The Fibre First Diet: How simply reordering your favourite foods effortlessly trims your waistline and wards off disease.* Primal Living.

If you enjoy pasta or rice-based meals, then you can adapt them to use vegetable alternatives – invest in a spiraliser to make leek of courgette 'spaghetti' to enjoy with your Bolognese sauce instead of pasta. If you love takeaway curries, you can still enjoy many of these dishes, although be aware that some may contain sugar. Instead of having rice with a curry, try curried mixed vegetables or non-starchy sides such as saag bhaji or cauliflower bhaji, or a bed of shredded lettuce. Try to consciously (re)train your mind and stomach to believe that curries don't have to be served with rice or chapattis. Some people make cauliflower 'rice' by stir-frying grated cauliflower. And instead of mashed potato on shepherd's pie, try mashed celeriac or cauliflower – they have only a fraction of the carbohydrate found in potato.

I suggest that you try to manage without desserts; if you eat a good main meal following the above guidelines, your body won't need a dessert. If you do fancy one, though, then berries with full-fat Greek yoghurt or crème fraiche are all very tasty, low-carb options. If you are having a special meal, then there are several low-carb dessert recipes available. Emma Porter at thelowcarbkitchen.co.uk has a recipe for a delicious chocolate mousse made with coconut milk or whipped cream and 90% dark chocolate. She also has recipes for low-carb crackers if you prefer cheese after a meal. Alternatively, eat cheese with celery instead of crackers.

Step 6: Watch what you drink

We have already discussed the need to reduce sugar in soft drinks and hot drinks. But what about alcohol? The NHS recommendation is to limit intake to 14 units a week or less. However, it is important to be aware that alcohol is very efficient at filling the liver with fat, which is one of the key steps in the obesity disease process. Alcohol is also very high in calories. So if you want to lose weight, especially if you drink more than 14 units a week, reducing your intake will certainly help. Some people choose to stop drinking alcohol altogether for a while as part of their journey to improved health.

If you drink alcohol, then it is important to know what effect your drinks will have on your blood glucose and insulin levels. Since alcohol is produced by fermentation of sugar, then as a rough rule of thumb, the higher the alcohol content, the lower the sugar content. Therefore, most spirits that are high in alcohol have no sugar in them. Dry red or white wine has a low sugar content and should not adversely affect your glucose levels, especially if drunk with a meal. Beer contains carbohydrate, and so I generally advise beer drinkers to think of beer as like any other carb-containing food and avoid drinking large quantities. The highest sugar levels are found in cider, sweet liqueurs, alcopops and some low-alcohol wines and beers, and these are best avoided altogether.

Change your diet before you start injections

I recommend that you make changes to your diet by following these steps as soon as you have committed yourself to trying to lose weight, and ideally before you start weight-loss injections. Reducing carbohydrates is one way of minimising the gut-related side effects of the injections (see Chapter 7). It also reduces the likelihood that the injections will increase insulin secretion after your meals, which in turn will make it more difficult for you to lose weight.

Most people find that their appetite reduces significantly when they start injections – this is part of how they work. But it is very important to ensure that you eat enough protein to minimise muscle loss. Therefore, please start to make changes to your diet, especially reducing carbohydrates and prioritising protein, **before** you start injections. This is discussed in more detail in Chapter 8.

Chapter 4

What kinds of exercise should I do while on weight-loss injections?

A lot of my overweight patients tell me they are overweight because they do not exercise enough, and they are often surprised when I tell them that exercise itself is unlikely to help them lose weight. Losing weight requires making the changes to your diet we have discussed.

Exercise is great for your heart and for building muscle strength, and later in this chapter I will describe some simple exercises you can do to build up your muscle bulk. It is also great for mental health and wellbeing. But it is not great for losing weight. And for people who are very overweight, the wrong type of exercise can pose a real risk of injury.

That's why I don't focus on exercise when I speak to people who want to lose weight. Too many people have negative connotations around exercise: failure, pain, Lycra, having to go to a gym, embarrassment about body image in the changing room, and so on. Consequently, people are usually very happy when I say 'Don't exercise! Walk instead.' And then I add 'Not a brisk walk; just a walk.' If a patient is unable to walk, I recommend that they move as much as possible using chair-based exercises. Any physical activity will do.

Back in the 1950s, research showed that people who walked as part of their job were healthier than those who sat down all day. One famous study looked at the health of two groups of workers on London buses: drivers (who spent several hours sitting behind the steering wheel) and conductors (whose job was to sell tickets to passengers, so they moved along the rows of seats and up and down the stairs all day long). The study also looked at postmen, who spent much of their day walking to deliver mail, and telephone switchboard operators who, like bus drivers, were seated during their working hours. They found that more active workers (postmen and bus conductors) had lower death rates from heart disease than their less active colleagues.[18]

More recently, the beneficial effects of physical activity on metabolic health were emphasised by a study from Denmark, in which active healthy volunteers were persuaded to reduce their activity from over 10,000 steps a day to less than 1,500.

---

18 Morris JN, Heady JA, et al. 'Coronary heart disease and physical activity at work.' *Lancet*, 1953, 1053–57.

After only two weeks they had higher blood insulin levels and a significant increase in abdominal fat,[19] both precursors to the development of Type 2 diabetes. So you can see that walking is good for metabolic health.

Walk your way to better health

But sitting down is not good for you. In one study, over 500 adults were asked to wear an accelerometer – a wearable device that measures activity levels. They also had various other measurements performed to assess their overall metabolic health. The accelerometers were analysed to determine how long they were inactive. The study concluded that the longer they sat down each day, the higher the level of insulin in their blood and the worse their insulin resistance. This inactive time was also associated with an increase in waist circumference of nearly 2 cm (about 0.75 of an inch) and with a reduction in healthy HDL cholesterol – both known consequences of insulin resistance.[20] This suggests that the more time we spend sitting down, the more likely we are

---

19 Olsen RH, et al. 'Metabolic responses to reduced daily steps in healthy nonexercising men.' *JAMA*, 2008, 299: 1261.
20 Healy GN, Dunstan DW, et al. 'Breaks in sedentary time: Beneficial associations with metabolic risk.' *Diabetes Care*, 2008, 31(4): 661–66.

to develop Type 2 diabetes. Indeed, this was the conclusion of a meta-analysis of a number of studies that looked at the effect of time spent watching TV on people's health. This showed that, on average, for every two hours spent watching television each day, the risk of developing Type 2 diabetes increased by 20%, and the risk of death from all causes increased by 13%. Incredibly, people who spent five hours a day watching television had a 50% increased risk of developing Type 2 diabetes.[21] The same likely applies to people who sit behind a screen all day at work.

As Type 2 diabetes is part of the obesity disease process, my advice to anyone who wants to lose weight is to **move more and to sit less**.

Walking is the ideal physical activity. It is free, does not require any special equipment, and is, lest we forget, a very useful form of transport. My focus is not on 'going out for a walk' – unless you are predominantly based at home – as that requires you to make the time to fit a walk into your daily routine. Rather, I encourage everyone to build walking into their daily routine. Here are some suggestions:

---

[21] Grøntved A, Hu FB. 'Television viewing and risk of Type 2 diabetes, cardiovascular disease, and all-cause mortality: A meta-analysis.' *JAMA*, 2011, 305(23): 2448–55.

A Guide to Weight Loss Injections

- If you use the bus, tram or Underground (metro or subway), get off at least one stop before you need to, so that you walk part of your journey.
- If you're driving somewhere, find a place to park a few hundred metres from where you need to be.
- If you're shopping at a supermarket or other store with a large car park, park as far away from the store entrance as you can.
- Choose to walk or cycle rather than use a car for any trips less than 2 km (1.5 miles).
- Use stairs rather than lifts or escalators.

If you are not used to walking, then I recommend that you choose one or two of these changes and give them a try. Remember, you don't have to walk briskly; walking at any speed is better than not walking at all. If you are overweight, then your knees or hips may ache to start with. But as you lose weight, these aches and pains should ease.

You might then try going out for a walk after lunch or your evening meal, as a way to use up the energy from the meal and minimise the rise in blood glucose that otherwise might occur. Even a fifteen-minute walk can help keep your blood glucose level stable after a meal.

The more you walk, the more your strength will improve and the easier and more enjoyable you will find it. Just a short walk significantly increases brain activity – and promotes a feeling of wellbeing. Research has shown that being in green spaces also improves health and wellbeing. That doesn't have to mean a walk in the country; it could be in a town park, or along a riverbank or even a tree-lined street, so if you can include these on your walking route, then you will gain an added benefit.

Sit down less

If my first message concerning physical activity is to walk more, my second is to sit down less – specifically, to try to **avoid sitting for longer than an hour at a time**. So many of us spend several hours each day, whether at work or at home, sitting in front of a screen, whether a television or a computer. Again, this is a huge change from a few decades ago. Anyone aged over forty will remember a time when most homes did not possess a computer, and anyone over thirty will remember a time when a mobile phone pretty much only made phone calls. The advent of laptops, smartphones and the internet mean that for many of us, work, play, shopping and socialising can all be done from the sofa, where we can spend hours on end, sitting, slouching or lying down. This is called sedentary time, and it is bad for our health.

A Guide to Weight Loss Injections

If watching more television increases the risk of Type 2 diabetes, then you would hope that reducing the amount of time you spend watching television would have the opposite effect. Support for this comes from a small study from the USA in which a group of thirty-six overweight people (with a BMI of between 25 and 50), who watched TV on average for three hours each day, were randomly split into a control group and an intervention group. The intervention group were asked to reduce their television viewing time by 50%. After three weeks, this group were found to have significantly increased their energy expenditure (measured using an accelerometer) and to have lost some weight.[22]

Even if you don't watch television, modern life means that long periods of sedentary time are inevitable for many of us – for example, people whose jobs involve driving or sitting at a desk. If this is you, what can you do to preserve your health? Studies have looked at the effect of 'breaks' in sedentary time. Research has shown that people who interrupted their sedentary time, even for only a minute, reduced their waist circumference, body weight and blood glucose levels,

---

22 Otten JJ, Jones KE, et al. 'Effects of television viewing reduction on energy intake and expenditure in overweight and obese adults.' Arch. Intern. Med., 2009, 169(22): 2109–15.

but people who did not interrupt their seated time did not.[23] There are several possible reasons for this, including the fact that the act of standing, even for a short time, uses significantly more energy than sitting down. I explain this using an analogy with a computer. If you do not use your computer for a certain length of time, it goes into sleep mode. That is, it is still on, but the screen has switched off and the processors have stopped processing and the fans have stopped whirring, in order to conserve energy. In the same way, if we do not use our body for a period, our metabolism goes into a sort of sleep mode, and slows down to use only enough energy to keep things ticking over. As a result, blood glucose levels rise and the energy saved is stored as fat in the liver – hence the increased waist circumference. The simple act of standing up has a similar effect to moving your computer's mouse: it wakes up your body, which starts operating again at full speed, consuming more energy as it does.

Take regular breaks if you sit all day

Try to avoid sitting down for longer than an hour. This means that if you are sitting at work all day, at your desk or in

---

23 Cooper RS, Sebire S, et al. 'Sedentary time, breaks in sedentary time and metabolic variables in people with newly diagnosed Type 2 diabetes.' *Diabetologia*, 2012, 55: 589–99.

a meeting, or in front of the TV at home, remind yourself to stand up at least once an hour and walk around for a couple of minutes before sitting down again and continuing to do what you were doing. You don't have to leave the room – although if you do venture outside for a couple of minutes, it will boost your system in other ways as well. Many people set their watch or their phone to buzz every hour to remind them to get up. At work, I suggest that people make their office as *inefficient* as possible, so that the printer or filing cabinet are not right next to their desk. Using a standing desk, or a desk that can be adjusted so you can work at it while standing, is a good way to reduce sitting time. Or use an under-desk exercise bike to move while you are working. Better still, incorporate some specific exercises into your daily routine, as discussed later in this chapter.

As I said earlier, many of my patients are delighted when I say 'Don't exercise, don't even think of joining a gym, simply walk more and sit less', but as they start to lose weight they find they can walk further without any aches and pains or shortness of breath. They feel healthier and better about themselves, and many choose to become more adventurous: they might dig out an old bike to rediscover how much they once enjoyed cycling, or they may join a local community run (such as Parkrun), knowing that it is perfectly okay to walk or to stop/start. No one is judging. Other initiatives include Couch to 5K (C25K), an exercise plan that gradually progresses from beginner running towards a 5-kilometre run over nine weeks. There are also walking football and walking netball, created to enable people to enjoy the games they used to love playing, but at a walking pace.

I mentioned earlier that exercise is good for overall health, and as you lose weight and become more mobile, you may find yourself wanting to begin a regime of more intensive exercise or join a gym or an exercise class. All exercise is good, provided you don't get over-ambitious and risk injuring yourself. Do whatever you find enjoyable! If you enjoy the exercise you do, you are more likely to keep it up.

Build muscle strength

Earlier, I mentioned that when people lose weight, there is a risk that they will lose muscle mass rather than fat, and I recently met someone who had direct experience of this. He had a DEXA scan that measured his body composition, and was advised to increase his protein intake and to do strength-training exercises to build his muscle mass while aiming to lose weight. He didn't follow this advice, and failed to lose weight. As the date of the follow-up scan approached, he went on a crash diet and was delighted to lose over 5 kg in weight. Delighted, that is, until the scan showed that of the 5 kg he had lost, 4 kg was muscle and only 1 kg was fat.

A Guide to Weight Loss Injections

All weight-loss diets involve losing some muscle as well as fat, and losing weight with injections is no different. But since they can lead to a lot of weight loss, there is the risk that the loss of muscle could pose problems, especially as we get older, when muscle mass begins to reduce naturally. So when a patient starts a weight-loss injection, I recommend some simple strength training, along with a good protein intake, to minimise such muscle loss.

I can testify to the benefits of strength training. Now well into my sixties, I have suffered from joint pain since early adulthood, when a virus led to inflammatory arthritis that affected many of my joints. Over the last few years, I have begun to experience severe knee and hip pain. Scans showed I had developed moderately severe osteoarthritis, possibly triggered by the virus I'd had years ago. I also began to experience lower back pain, particularly after carrying my young grandchildren, and I was aware that the strength in my arms was reducing as the muscles were shrinking. My legs remained quite strong, as I walk and cycle a reasonable amount. I sought the advice of a physiotherapist, who recommended that while I cannot undo the damage already done to my joints, I can relieve the symptoms by building up the strength of the muscles around the joints and thereby stabilising them. In the past I have joined a gym, but found that some exercises made my symptoms worse. This emphasises the importance of having an exercise programme tailored to your specific needs, especially if you have health issues. So I looked for someone who could give me insightful advice and came across James Beeson. James learned his trade in the army and devised a programme to suit my needs. Within a few weeks, my back pain, knee pain and hip pain had all improved significantly and I was able to walk further without limping. I gained about 2 kg in weight, and while I haven't had DEXA scans to show that the weight gained is muscle, my previously rather feeble muscles are no longer looking quite so feeble so I know at least some of the extra weight is due to increased muscle mass. As many of my patients who are overweight also experience joint pain, they will also benefit from similar strength-training exercises both to reduce pain and to ensure that, as they lose weight, they build up their muscle mass as much as possible. It's also important to do the right exercises, especially if your mobility is limited by carrying excess weight. No one wants to make things worse. I asked James to list some simple exercises that he would recommend to someone who is overweight and who has not exercised for many years. They can all be done at home without special equipment, and I have included some here.

James emphasises the importance of starting with easy exercises and building them into your routine: consistency is key to building up your muscles. If at the moment you rarely walk, he suggests starting by getting up and walking for five minutes as many times during the day as you can manage.

A Guide to Weight Loss Injections

This can be done indoors. When you feel you are able, go for a longer walk outside once or twice a day, aiming for fifteen minutes duration initially. This in itself will help increase your exercise capacity, and you will then be able to increase the length of the walk quite easily. James recommends you then start with three strength-training exercises: squats, hinges and planks.

Squats

When you first do this, support yourself by holding on to the edge of your kitchen worktop, with your hands about 2 feet (60 cm) apart. Stand with your feet in line with your shoulders about 18 inches (45 cm) apart and relax your hips, knees and ankles. Keeping your feet flat on the ground and your back as straight as you can, gently lower your hips as if you were going to sit in a chair. Bend your knees to lower your bottom as far as you can comfortably without losing your balance, but not lower than your knees. Then straighten your legs back to the standing position, using your arms to help push yourself up if necessary. The first time you do this, you might only manage it once or twice. It really doesn't matter. This is the start of your journey to bring new life back into your muscles and joints. Remember, if you have been carrying excess weight for years, it will be your hips and knees that have suffered the most – so be gentle on them!

Try this every day and gradually build up until you can do this five times in a row. As your muscles get stronger, you can then try the same exercise but, instead of holding on to your kitchen worktop, clasp your hands together in front of you, so you are relying on your leg muscles alone to get back up again. Squats help to build strength in the muscles in your legs and bottom, and support the hip and knee joints, making it easier for you to stand up, sit down and get in and out of a car, for example.

Hinges

This is a great exercise to strengthen core muscles in your lower back and upper legs. It involves pushing your hips backwards, while keeping your back relatively straight, a bit like the position a ski jumper adopts as they speed along the slope before take-off – knees slightly bent and leaning forward at the hips (remember Eddie the Eagle?). To do this, stand with your feet in line with your shoulders and relax your knees and hips. Tighten your tummy muscles and push your hips backwards, as if you are sitting back into a chair, while moving your upper body forward to about 45 degrees, keeping your back straight. Then reverse the movement by squeezing your glutes (bum cheeks) and pushing your feet into the floor and your hips forward to stand upright again. Again, aim to build up so that you do this five times each day.

A Guide to Weight Loss Injections

Straight-arm planks

Once you have mastered the above exercises, you can add the straight-arm plank. This is a bit more challenging, as it involves getting down on all fours on the floor. This exercise is great for strengthening your stomach muscles as well as your back and glutes. It can help improve your overall posture and upper body strength. To start, get down onto all fours and make sure your hands are directly under your shoulders. Straighten one leg and then the other, lifting your knees off the ground so that your body is in a straight line from your head to your heels. Squeeze your tummy muscles and your bum and hold this position for as long as you can, then lower your knees to the ground again. You might only manage to hold the plank position for a few seconds to start with, but with practice, you should be able to gradually increase the time you can hold the position.

James has made some videos to explain these and other exercises, which you can view using this link: www.jamesbeesonfitness.com

These exercises are specifically designed to build up your muscle bulk and to minimise loss of muscle as you lose weight. They should be done in addition to walking, which has all the benefits we discussed earlier. However, if walking is difficult for you, then try cycling on an exercise bike to get your legs moving in a non-weight-bearing way.

As you strengthen your muscles and lose weight, you will find the exercises become easier for you. You may then feel able to join an exercise class (or yoga or Pilates), which will help to strengthen your core and limb muscles. As you lose weight, your energy levels will increase and you may even find yourself enjoying walking, cycling or even playing a team sport that you stopped participating in years ago.

Chapter 5

Wegovy and Mounjaro

In Chapter 2 we used insulin as an example of a hormone that is produced in one part of the body – the pancreas – and has effects in other organs, including the liver and muscles. Wegovy and Mounjaro, the two weight-loss injections available in the UK, increase the activity of another, less well-known hormone called glucagon-like peptide-1 (GLP-1 for short). GLP-1 is produced in the intestines in response to food intake. It is a very busy molecule, with the following actions:

- It increases the release of insulin and inhibits the release of glucagon in the pancreas. This ensures that glucose from the meal is taken up into cells for energy or stored for later use.
- It slows the emptying of the stomach, so food stays in the stomach for longer, ensuring complete digestion but crucially also increasing satiety, so that you feel fuller for longer after a meal.

- It sends signals to the brain regions involved in hunger regulation, reducing appetite and the desire to eat.

GLP-1 was discovered in the 1980s during research on intestinal hormones. It's a part of a larger molecule, proglucagon, a protein consisting of 160 amino acids. Its significant role in regulating glucose levels led to interest in its potential for treating Type 2 diabetes. In the 1990s drug companies began to develop synthetic GLP-1 receptor agonists (a substance which initiates a physiological response when combined with a receptor). These agents were designed to mimic the effects of natural GLP-1, especially its ability to enhance insulin secretion and lower blood glucose levels. The first such agent, exenatide, was derived from the saliva of the Gila monster and entered clinical testing for diabetes. It was launched for use in 2007. During clinical trials of GLP-1 agonists for diabetes treatment, researchers noticed that these drugs also led to weight loss in patients, an effect that had not been anticipated. This sparked interest in exploring the potential of GLP-1 receptor agonists as treatments for obesity. In the mid-2000s studies began to show that drugs such as exenatide and liraglutide could reduce body weight in patients without diabetes, leading to excitement within the medical community. The next GLP-1 agonist was liraglutide, a modified version of GLP-1. It was shown to produce more significant weight loss than exenatide. A pivotal study, the SCALE trial, demonstrated that liraglutide reduced body weight by about 5–10% over the course of a year in individuals with obesity.[24]

In 2015, liraglutide (marketed as Saxenda) was approved by the European Medicines Agency and launched in the UK in 2017. Within the NHS, its use was restricted to people with obesity and prediabetes and at increased risk of cardiovascular disease. It could only be prescribed by specialist weight management services. These limitations mean that it did not take off to the same extent as its descendants – Wegovy and Mounjaro. It was, however, the first GLP-1 agonist licensed explicitly for weight loss, rather than as a diabetes treatment. Clinical studies confirmed that liraglutide was well tolerated, with the most common side effects being nausea and vomiting. Most patients experienced weight loss of between 5–10%.

Further research by the drug company Novo Nordisk in Denmark led to the development of semaglutide. It was launched in the UK in early 2019 as Ozempic, a treatment for Type 2 diabetes. In 2023 it was launched for the management of obesity under the tradename Wegovy. It had a stronger effect than liraglutide, and in trials participants lost an average of 15–20% of their body weight, which was far

---

[24] Pi-Sunyer X, et al. 'A randomized, controlled trial of 3.0 mg of liraglutide in weight management.' *N. Engl. J. Med.*, 2015, 373: 11–22.

greater than had been observed with any other anti-obesity medication.[25]

Further research and clinical experience have determined that Wegovy promotes weight loss in different ways. Its main action is to increase feelings of satiety and reducing hunger. It does this by slowing gastric emptying, which prolongs the sensation of fullness after eating, and by acting on the hypothalamus in the brain to limit appetite and food intake. This is particularly important for patients with obesity, who often experience reduced satiety and may be prone to overeating. There is also some evidence that it can increase the burning of fat for energy, thus reducing fat stores in the liver and other organs. This has the added benefit of reducing insulin resistance and helping to reverse the obesity disease process, described in Chapter 2. Its effects on the release of insulin and glucagon from the pancreas are most important for people with diabetes. However, the overall impact of these actions is to reduce glucose levels after meals, thus reducing high insulin levels, which is important in reducing fat stores in people with obesity, even if they do not have diabetes.

---

[25] Wilding J, et al. 'Once-weekly semaglutide in adults with overweight or obesity.' *N. Engl. J. Med.*, 2021, 384: 989–1002.

GLP-1 agonists also influence other hormones involved in appetite regulation. For example, they suppress the release of ghrelin, a hormone that stimulates hunger, while increasing the release of peptide YY, another gut hormone that reduces hunger. This complex interaction between different hormones helps make it easier for patients to manage their appetite.

Finally, there is some evidence that GLP-1 agonists affect the brain's reward pathways, which are involved in the motivation to eat and the pleasure derived from food. These drugs may alter how the brain perceives food-related rewards. This can help reduce food cravings and compulsive eating, which are experienced by many people living with obesity. Using the injections can help reduce what has become known as 'food noise'. Food noise refers to constantly thinking about food. It has been described as incessant mental chatter, making us crave food even when our bodies do not need it. Food noise is driven by emotional and psychological factors, such as stress, anxiety or boredom.

Mounjaro

The newest weight-loss drug is tirzepatide, launched in the UK in February 2024 by Eli Lilly under the brand name Mounjaro. Like Wegovy, it is a GLP-1 agonist with the same effects. It has additional effects as it also activates GIP (gastric inhibitory polypeptide) receptors in the gut. Like GLP-1, GIP increases insulin release from the pancreas after meals. This effect is stronger in individuals who are insulin resistant, such as those with Type 2 diabetes or obesity. At the same time, GIP improves insulin sensitivity in muscle and fat cells, thus reducing insulin resistance.

GIP appears to have a stronger effect than GLP-1 in promoting the breakdown of fat. Its role in reducing appetite is less well understood than GLP-1s, but there is evidence that activating the GIP receptor in combination with GLP-1 may contribute to enhanced satiety and weight loss. Some studies suggest that GIP may prolong the appetite effects of GLP-1 so that they do not reduce over time.

The 'dual action' of Mounjaro mean that it can promote greater weight loss than Wegovy. It has shown remarkable results in clinical trials for weight loss, which in some studies was over 20% after one year of treatment.[26] In the UK Mounjaro is available as a weight-loss treatment for people with or without diabetes.

---

[26] Jastreboff A, et al. 'Tirzepatide once weekly for the treatment of obesity.' *N. Engl. J. Med.*, 2022, 387: 205–16.

How to access Wegovy or Mounjaro

In the UK, EU and USA, Wegovy has been licensed for use as a treatment of obesity in people with a BMI of 30 or above, or 27 or above in people with weight-related health problems.

Within the UK, these medications are available via the NHS, according to the recommendations of the National Institute for Health and Care Excellence (NICE). According to NICE, Wegovy is recommended as an option for weight management, including weight loss and weight maintenance, alongside a reduced-calorie diet and increased physical activity in adults. It is recommended for people with a BMI of at least 30 (27.5 in people from Asian, Middle Eastern, Black African or African-Caribbean family backgrounds) who have at least one weight-related condition. NICE states that Wegovy can only be provided via a specialist weight management service and for a maximum duration of two years.

Interestingly, NICE takes a different view on Mounjaro in three important respects:

- It is only recommended for people with a BMI of 35 or higher (32.5 in people from other ethnic groups) and a weight-related condition.

- It can be prescribed by a primary care professional (such as a GP) and not just a specialist service.
- There is no time limit for its use.

In the first year of implementation (2025–26), the NHS is restricting Mounjaro to people with a BMI of over 40, who also have four of the following associated weight-related health conditions: high blood pressure, high cholesterol level, obstructive sleep apnoea, cardiovascular disease or Type 2 diabetes. Over the following years, this will change to include people with a BMI over 35 and/or three associated health conditions.

For both drugs, it is recommended that people who do not lose at least 5% of their body weight in the first six months stop treatment.

While Mounjaro should be restricted to people with more severe obesity, NICE recommends that it should be more easily accessible and for a longer duration than Wegovy. I can see no logical reason for this difference and suspect that, in time, NICE will also recommend that Wegovy is made more widely accessible. It is important to be aware that simply because NICE makes a recommendation, it does not mean that your GP will be able to prescribe the drug, as each local health authority (now known as Integrated Care Boards) must decide how to interpret and implement NICE recommendations. Obesity treatments are to be phased in over twelve years, and that means that many people will have a long wait to access them via the NHS.

These restrictions in the UK mean that a lot of people turn to private providers to access the drugs. **It is important that this is done under medical supervision and follow-up**, to quickly identify and manage side effects (see Chapter 7) and to provide appropriate lifestyle advice. Participants in the research studies of these medications received lifestyle advice in addition to the medications, and the regulations governing their use stipulate that the drugs should be used as part of a weight-loss management strategy. There are several online pharmacies that offer Wegovy and Mounjaro following a basic assessment based on data you provide them. While they can provide the medications, I am not aware of any that provide the recommended lifestyle advice or follow-up. Unsurprisingly, some people have found a way around the assessment process, and alarming reports have emerged over the past few years about how people have bought them from online pharmacies, despite not meeting the criteria for prescription within their licence. This includes people with eating disorders who are not obese being able to access the drugs to promote severe weight loss. As a result, it is anticipated that the rules will be strengthened to prevent such abuse.

Reports have also emerged of unscrupulous websites that sell fake products. Sometimes these contain insulin, which is particularly dangerous as it can cause dangerously low blood glucose levels, especially in someone who does not have diabetes or who is taking other diabetes medications.

If you do meet the criteria for using weight-loss injections, then purchasing the drugs from an online pharmacy can be appropriate, provided you are fully aware of the possible risks and side effects that can be associated with taking them and that you can access medical help if needed. Private clinics are not bound by NICE guidance, but the drugs must be prescribed in accordance with their licence, which in both cases makes provision for them to be used in people with a BMI of 30 or above, or a BMI of 27 or more in people who have an additional weight-related condition. At the time of writing, Wegovy costs between £100 and £200 per month, and Mounjaro between £170 and £300, depending on the dose required.

Both medications are given by subcutaneous injection, and start at a low dose which is then gradually increased as required. In the UK, both are dispensed using an injection pen device that contains four doses, and each pen is supplied with four needles (one for each dose). In the USA, each pen has a needle already attached and is used for a single dose. The needles are very fine and just 4 mm long (about 1/6 of an inch). For most people the injections are entirely painless. I promise.

A Guide to Weight Loss Injections

You should be given full instructions about how to use the pens to inject the drug you are prescribed. As the finer details will vary, I will not cover these in detail here. The drugs need to be injected into the fat below the skin in the abdomen (at least 5 cm from your belly button), thigh or upper arm. Ideally, they should be given on the same day each week, at a time of day that suits you. They do not need to be given with food. It is important that the pens are stored in the fridge before use (ideally at 2–8°C). Do not freeze them! Used needles should be deposited in a sharps bin that must be disposed of safely, according to the arrangements where you live.

Wegovy is started at a dose of 0.25 mg, and Mounjaro at 2.5 mg. The manufacturers of both drugs recommend that users move to a higher dose after four weeks, according to the schedule in Table 5.1.

Table 5.1. Dosage of Wegovy and Mounjaro over time.

	Wegovy	Mounjaro
Weeks 1–4	0.25 mg	2.5 mg
Weeks 5–8	0.5 mg	5 mg
Weeks 9–12	1 mg	7.5 mg
Weeks 13–16	1.7 mg	10 mg
Weeks 17–20	2.4 mg	12.5 mg
Week 20 onwards	2.4 mg	15 mg

This gradual stepwise dose increase is designed to help your body get used to the effects of the drug, and to reduce the likelihood of side effects. The most common initial side effect is nausea, and this alone can reduce your appetite very significantly. It is usually transient, lasting for a day or two after each injection, and generally gets easier with each injection. It may return, however, as you increase the dose. Some people experience vomiting and/or diarrhoea, particularly after eating certain foods. If this occurs, I recommend you make a note of the foods that caused the problem and avoid them in future or try a much smaller portion, especially if they are fatty foods. If you experience side effects, I generally advise not to increase the dose, and to consider reducing to the previous dose until the side effects settle down. In my practice, I do not recommend automatically increasing the dose every four weeks; if you are seeing benefits such as reduced appetite and weight loss on a low dose, I suggest remaining on that dose for as long as you can. I am finding, along with other doctors, that so-called microdosing can be very effective and in some cases people can gain benefit from taking half the standard starting dose. Not only will this minimise the risk of side effects, it also significantly reduces the cost of the treatment. Unfortunately, many online pharmacies seem to automatically recommend an increase in dose every four weeks: since they provide no clinical supervision, this can be dangerous if someone is experiencing side effects on the lower dose.

Children

It is a sad reflection of our society that obesity rates are rising among children. Wegovy is licensed for use by children from the age of twelve if their BMI is in the 95th centile or more (that is, they weigh more than 95% of all children of their age) and their body weight is above 60 kg. The recommended dosing is the same as for adults, starting at 0.25 mg per week and increasing to a maximum of 2.4 mg weekly. A clinical trial that compared Wegovy to a placebo (a dummy injection) for sixty-eight weeks in a group of adolescents showed that it was associated with significant weight loss.[27] Their average age was 15.5 years and body weight before treatment was 110 kg (BMI 37.7), indicating significant obesity. They lost an average of 15.3 kg body weight and 12.7 cm from their waist. Although not discussed in the research paper, the data showed that around 10% of the study participants actually gained weight while supposedly taking the injections.

---

27 Weghuber D, et al. 'Once-weekly semaglutide in adolescents with obesity.' *N. Engl. J. Med.*, 2022, 387: 2245–57.

Their cholesterol level and blood pressure also reduced. In the placebo group, the average weight loss was 2.4 kg. Gut side effects (nausea, vomiting and diarrhoea) occurred in 62% of the youngsters taking Wegovy, mostly as the dose was being increased. These were generally mild and lasted two to three days: however, 1 in 20 stopped the treatment because of these effects. More serious side effects such as gallstones occurred in five of those taking Wegovy, compared to none in the placebo group This study showed that most of the teenagers were able to tolerate the treatment, which was far more effective in helping weight loss than previous GLP-1 agonists such as liraglutide. The study also showed weight gain in the few weeks after treatment was stopped, and we do not know how much weight the participants have since regained. Unlike Wegovy, Mounjaro is not licensed for use by children. Trulicity (dulaglutide) has a weaker effect and is licensed for use in children from the age of ten.

Chapter 6
Other benefits of weight-loss injections

In the years since GLP-1 agonists have been used as a treatment for diabetes, a lot of evidence has accumulated on how they are also beneficial to other aspects of health. This is not altogether surprising, as being overweight impacts so many aspects of health, but it is encouraging that these treatments have the potential to improve several weight-related problems. To date, there is much less evidence for Mounjaro, as it is so much newer, but it would be expected to have similar benefits.

Some of the benefits arise directly from losing weight and are quite obvious. For example, back, hip and knee pain will likely improve significantly in someone who loses a lot of weight. Sleep problems, especially sleep apnoea, can also be expected to improve, as can symptoms related to oesophageal reflux. In people with diabetes, many symptoms associated with high glucose levels will improve.

There are in addition a number of less direct benefits that we will discuss in this chapter. These include positive effects on the heart, kidney, liver and brain. We will also look at the potential of these drugs in improving fertility, reducing cancer risk and in managing addictions.

The heart

All new diabetes drugs must undergo research to identify the impact they have on heart health. These are known as cardiovascular outcomes trials (CVOTs), and they came about following the sorry story of a drug called rosiglitazone that was licensed for the management of diabetes in 1999; it then had to be withdrawn as it was shown to increase the risk of heart disease. The CVOTs for GLP-1 agonists have consistently demonstrated that these medications are actually very good for the heart. Semaglutide (the active ingredient in Wegovy) was studied in the SUSTAIN-6 trial and showed that it was associated with a 26% reduction in major cardiovascular events (which includes stroke as well as heart attacks).[28] These studies were done in people with Type 2 diabetes. It is well established that reducing glucose levels

---

28 Marso S, et al. 'Semaglutide and cardiovascular outcomes in patients with Type 2 diabetes.' *N. Engl. J. Med.*, 2016, 375: 1834–44.

is good for the heart, so it would be expected that a diabetes drug that reduces glucose levels would be beneficial. However, it appears that GLP-1 agonists have other specific actions on the heart, as it has been identified that GLP-1 receptors are found in heart muscle cells and the endothelial cells that line blood vessels. In the heart muscle, GLP-1 increases the entry of glucose into the cells, where is used as fuel. It also reduces cell damage (apoptosis). Together these effects protect heart function. Research published in October 2025 showed that people who took Wegovy as a treatment for obesity had a reduced risk of a cardiovascular event, as might be expected. However, the reduction in risk was not dependent on the amount of weight lost, supporting the idea that the drug has additional effects that protect the heart, beyond the effect of weight loss.[29]

In blood vessels, GLP-1 stimulates the production of nitric oxide (NO). NO is a vasodilator that opens the blood vessels and improves blood flow through them. This improves blood flow in the coronary arteries that supply the heart muscle. More generally, it helps to reduce blood pressure. These

---

[29] Deanfield J, et al. 'Semaglutide and cardiovascular outcomes by baseline and changes in adiposity measurements: A prespecified analysis of the SELECT trial.' Lancet, 2025. https://doi.org/10.1016/S0140-6736(25)01375-3

effects thus help reverse the effect of high insulin levels in constricting blood vessels.

The kidneys

The benefits of GLP-1 agonists in reducing body weight and blood pressure and improving blood flow are also good for the kidneys. In studies in people with diabetes, GLP-1 agonists slowed down the decline in kidney function that had previously occurred, and reduced the leakage of protein into the urine due to kidney damage. There is also evidence that these treatments reduce inflammation in the kidneys. These benefits have been shown with Mounjaro as well as Wegovy, and are likely to be seen in people without diabetes who take these medications for obesity.[30]

The liver

In Chapter 2 we discussed how excess fat is present in the livers of people with clinical obesity, and how this contributes to insulin resistance and many of the health problems

---

30 Alicic R, et al. 'Incretin Therapies for Patients with Type 2 Diabetes and Chronic Kidney Disease.' *J. Clin. Med.*, 2024, 13: 201–17.

associated with it. This accumulation of fat is known as metabolic dysfunction-associated steatotic liver disease (MASLD) and can lead to metabolic dysfunction-associated steatohepatitis (MASH) and even cirrhosis. GLP-1 agonists have been shown to protect the liver by improving hepatic mitochondrial function and insulin sensitivity.

They also reduce the accumulation of fat in the liver. Studies have shown that patients with MASH have reduced natural production of GLP-1 in the gut, suggesting that GLP-1 agonists could be an effective treatment for MASH. Both Wegovy and Mounjaro have been shown to improve MASH by reducing fat accumulation and inflammation in the liver.[31,32] Studies are currently under way to look in more detail at the effect of these treatments in improving MASH, to find out whether they can reduce scarring (fibrosis), which is the early stage of cirrhosis.

---

31 Mahapatra M, et al. 'Therapeutic potential of semaglutide, a newer GLP-1 receptor agonist, in abating obesity, non-alcoholic steatohepatitis and neurodegenerative diseases: A narrative review.' *Pharm. Res.*, 2022, 39: 1233–48.

32 Loomba R, et al. 'Tirzepatide for metabolic dysfunction-associated steatohepatitis with liver fibrosis.' *N. Engl. J. Med.*, 2024, 391: 299–310.

The brain

Earlier we saw how GLP-1 agonists reduce vascular events such as strokes. A stroke occurs when narrowing of one of the arteries in the brain causes damage to the area of the brain supplied by that artery. Strokes, like other vascular disease, are a common complication of the obesity disease process. They can be very severe, leading to unconsciousness and death, or relatively mild, causing a mild weakness in one part of the body that can recover over time.

Another brain disease associated with obesity is Alzheimer's disease or dementia. In this, memory and brain function are impaired, and it can also affect speech, behaviour and movement. Animal studies have shown promising results where semaglutide (Wegovy) reduced brain inflammation and led to improved movement.[33] They have also shown that Wegovy protects brain cells from injury and helps to reduce inflammation. Studies are currently under way to see if semaglutide can improve brain function in people with established dementia. It may be that by that stage, treatment will have only a limited effect: however, it is likely that

---

33 Du H, et al. 'The mechanism and efficacy of GLP-1 receptor agonists in the treatment of Alzheimer's disease.' *Front. Endocrinol.*, 2022. https://doi.org/10.3389/fendo.2022.1033479

treatment with Wegovy or Mounjaro for obesity will also help protect the brain from the development of dementia.

Cancer

In Chapter 2 we mentioned that obesity is associated with an increased risk of breast cancer, womb (uterus) cancer, bowel cancer, pancreatic cancer and liver cancer. It has been suggested that one of the benefits of treatments such as Wegovy and Mounjaro could be that it helps reduce this cancer risk. Much research has been conducted looking at the effect of these drugs on cancer cell lines. Beneficial effects have been demonstrated where the drugs reduced the proliferation of cells on their own, and also where they made cells more susceptible to anti-cancer chemotherapy treatments. Such effects have been observed with pancreas, breast, prostate, uterus, ovary and colon cancer cells.[34] Regardless of whether the drugs are developed for future use to treat cancer, these findings raise the possibility that they will help reduce the risk of these cancers in people who take them. However, concerns have also been raised about the potential for GLP-1

---

34 Wang J, et al. 'Differential risk of cancer associated with glucagon-like peptide-1 receptor agonists: Analysis of real-world databases.' *Endocr. Res.*, 2022, 47: 18–25.

agonists to increase the risk of some cancers. This will be discussed in more detail in Chapter 7.

Fertility

In Chapter 2, we described how polycystic ovary syndrome (PCOS) is a common condition in women, resulting from an imbalance of sex hormones in association with insulin resistance. This can lead to a relative excess of testosterone, which can lead to increased body hair and male-pattern scalp baldness. It also leads to infrequent or absent periods and infertility. Since GLP-1 agonists help to reduce insulin resistance, they have been studied as possible treatments for PCOS. In one study of 72 overweight women with PCOS who were treated with liraglutide (Saxenda) or a placebo for 26 weeks, treatment with liraglutide reduced body weight by over 5%, liver fat by 44% and testosterone level by 19%.[35] Other studies showed that liraglutide treatment helped reduce the size of ovaries that were enlarged because of cysts, and that it was effective as a preconception treatment in combination with metformin in increasing in vitro fertilisation (IVF) pregnancy rates. Clinical trials also showed that exenatide

---

35 Nylander M, et al. 'Effects of liraglutide on ovarian dysfunction in polycystic ovary syndrome: A randomized clinical trial.' *RBMO*, 2016. https://doi.org/10.1016/j.rbmo.2017.03.023

(Byetta) improved menstrual regularity and ovulation rate in women with PCOS, which directly translates to enhanced fertility.

Taken together, this research confirms that GLP-1 agonists have beneficial effects in reducing the hormonal imbalance and infertility that occurs in PCOS, in addition to weight-loss effects. However, there is evidence that GLP-1 agonists can be associated with complications during pregnancy, so it is essential that women in their reproductive years should be on effective contraception while on therapy.

Men living with obesity can also be affected by infertility because of an impact on the hormones that control testosterone levels and sperm production. Recent laboratory research has shown that the use of GLP-1 agonists improves sperm metabolism and motility. A clinical trial in men with obesity and reduced sperm count showed that treatment with liraglutide was associated with improvements in sperm count, erectile function and testosterone levels.[36] These changes are likely to be secondary to weight loss and improved insulin sensitivity, as seen in women with PCOS.

---

36 Varnum A. 'Impact of GLP-1 agonists on male reproductive health – a narrative review.' *Medicina*, 2024, 60: 50.

Addictions

A very interesting and perhaps unexpected side effect of using weight-loss injections has been that people report losing their interest in drinking alcohol. So much so, that the drinks industry is bracing itself for falling sales as more people use the medications. It has led to headlines such as 'Skinny jabs are turning slimmers teetotal – and drinks companies are feeling the loss'.[37] Users report that alcohol worsens the nausea they experience with the injections, or that the injections make hangovers worse. A lot of research has been done to explore the impact that GLP-1 agonists have on the brain, and in particular the reward centres that are activated by drinking alcohol or using drugs such as heroin or cocaine.

The nucleus accumbens (NAc) is a structure deep in the basal ganglia, one of the oldest parts of the brain in evolutionary terms. It plays an important role in processing reward and pleasure and is often considered the pleasure centre of the brain. It is highly influenced by dopamine, a neurotransmitter (a chemical connector between brain cells) that is critical in so-called reward pathways. Studies in mice have shown that GLP-1 agonists block the release of dopamine in this reward centre, so that they do not feel the expected reward or pleasure from drinking alcohol. Further studies

---

37 *The Observer*, 26 January 2025.

showed that GLP-1 treatment also reduced the motivation (in rats) to consume alcohol, when they are given a choice.[38] It also reduces withdrawal symptoms when they were denied alcohol, reducing the likelihood that they would consume alcohol when it was again available.

One study has looked at the use of exenatide as a treatment for people with alcohol use disorder. It showed significant changes in the reward centre in the brain associated with drinking alcohol. Furthermore, exenatide reduced heavy drinking in the subjects who were also obese. These fascinating insights are consistent with the known fact that GLP-1 acts in the brain to reduce appetite for food, and tally with the experience of people who use Wegovy: that their interest in and reward from alcohol has been reduced – bad news indeed for the drinks industry.

Ultra-processed food addiction is increasingly recognised as a reason why many people struggle to lose weight. Like other addictions, this is associated with intense cravings for addictive food and what has become known as 'food noise', as I mentioned previously. It was a new term to me when I began writing this book: I was introduced to it by a patient

---

38 Jerlhag E. 'The therapeutic potential of glucagon-like peptide-1 for persons with addictions based on findings from preclinical and clinical studies.' *Front. Pharmacol.*, 2023. https://doi.org/10.3389/fphar.2023.1063033

who was very obese and had been diagnosed with Type 2 diabetes. She was making great efforts to change her diet and requested Mounjaro to help switch off food noise, about which I knew very little. There is still no formal definition of food noise, but it refers generally to persistent and intrusive thoughts about food that can make it difficult to focus on other tasks or maintain a healthy relationship with eating. It is usually associated with constant cravings for certain foods (often UPFs) and is often seen in people who experience UPF addiction. It is likely to be related to the effect of such foods in activating the brain's reward pathways, making it harder to resist cravings.

The key to reducing food noise is to stop activating those reward pathways, and that means moving away from UPFs and to protein-rich real foods, as I described in Chapter 3. This, I recognise, is much easier said than done, especially if you are addicted to UPFs. I have now seen many patients who have used Wegovy or Mounjaro and found them very effective in reducing food noise, making it easier for them to focus on eating more healthily without constant cravings for unhealthy food.

Chapter 7

Side effects of weight-loss injections and how to manage them

Every single drug has side effects, and it is important to take these into account when considering starting a new medication. Weight-loss injections are no different. In recent years, an increasing number of news stories have detailed how weight-loss injections have caused all sorts of side effects, from the relatively trivial (such as no longer wanting to drink alcohol) to the fatal (such as cases of inflammation of the pancreas). In this chapter we will focus on the reported side effects and what can be done to minimise them. To begin with, we will look at the more serious side effects – and why *some* people should not start treatment with weight-loss injections, because of the risk of side effects.

Pancreatic disease

One of the biggest anxieties surrounding these medications is their effect on the pancreas, and in particular, that they can cause inflammation of the pancreas (pancreatitis). This is highlighted by tragic cases such as the nurse in the UK who developed pancreatitis and organ failure and died after taking only two injections of Mounjaro.[39] However, obesity itself is associated with an increased risk of pancreatitis, and in the clinical trials, similar numbers of cases of pancreatitis occurred in both the treatment and the control groups (who took dummy medication). In some studies, pancreatitis was slightly more common in the control group.[40] In the SUSTAIN 6 trial, for example, there were nine cases of acute pancreatitis in the treatment group and twelve in the control group.[41] Although there is no evidence of a strong link between the use of weight-loss injections and pancreatitis, it is generally advised that anyone with a history of pancreatitis should not take these medications.

---

39 https://www.bbc.co.uk/news/articles/cz6jg6nw2zeo
40 Smits MM, 'Safety of semaglutide.' *Front. Endocrinol.*, 2021, 12. https://doi.org/10.3389/fendo.2021.645563
41 Marso SP, et al. 'Semaglutide and cardiovascular outcomes in patients with Type 2 diabetes.' *N. Engl. J. Med.*, 2016, 375: 1834–44.

Thyroid cancer

There is also concern about these drugs increasing the risk of thyroid cancer. This was initially seen in studies on animals, in which the drugs led to an increased risk of a type of thyroid cancer called medullary carcinoma. This is a very rare type of thyroid cancer in any case, so it can be difficult to determine whether a particular medication increases the risk. In the clinical trials of Wegovy and Mounjaro, no increase in thyroid cancer was observed. While some studies of its use in clinical practice have shown a higher number of cases of thyroid cancer in people taking GLP-1 injections, detailed analysis has failed to establish a definite link.[42] The European Medicines Agency has recommended that weight-loss medications can be taken safely by people with thyroid conditions, apart from people with a personal or family history of medullary thyroid carcinoma, or a rare condition called MEN2 (multiple endocrine neoplasia type 2, in which medullary cancer occurs with other hormone-related conditions),

---

42 Espinosa De Ycaza AE, et al. 'Glucaogon-like peptide-1 receptor agonists and thyroid cancer: A narrative review.' *Thyroid*, 2025, 34: 403–18.

Pregnancy

Animal studies have shown that use of these drugs causes toxicity to the growing foetus, and these drugs must therefore **not be taken during pregnancy**. Women of childbearing age are therefore advised to use effective contraception while they are taking these medications, and for at least two months after stopping treatment. Animal studies also showed that Wegovy appears in breast milk, and so it should not be taken by any women who are breastfeeding. There is no information on the use of Mounjaro while breastfeeding, and so it is not advised.

Diabetic eye disease (retinopathy)

The use of weight-loss injections in people who have diabetic eye disease has shown an increased risk of deterioration in their eye condition. Specifically, one of the large studies of Wegovy showed an increased need for treatment of diabetic eye disease in people who took the medication.[43] It is well known that a rapid improvement in blood glucose levels can paradoxically worsen diabetic eye disease, and it is likely that

---

43 Sharma A, et al. 'Semaglutide and the risk of diabetic retinopathy – current perspective.' *Eye*, 2021, 36: 10–11.

this is the explanation for the worsening problems when using these medications, rather than an adverse effect of the drugs themselves. Nevertheless, people with active diabetic eye disease are advised not to use these medications. In certain cases, they can be used if the diabetic eye disease has settled down, but such cases require regular eye examinations to detect any deterioration in the diabetic eye disease while the patient takes the medication.

Gallstones

A number of studies have shown an increased risk of gallstones and gallbladder infections in people taking weight-loss injections; this has not been seen in people using other medications associated with weight loss. These drugs reduce the motility of the gut, and as the gallbladder is part of the gut, then one can easily appreciate how reducing contractions in the gallbladder could lead to bile not being emptied fully from the gallbladder and therefore increasing the risk of developing gallstones plus gallbladder infection. For this reason, people who have a history of gallstones may be advised not to take these medications.

Mental health

Some studies have shown that GLP-1 agonists are associated with an increased risk of mental health problems and an increase in suicidal thoughts, although this is extremely rare. If you are experiencing suicidal thoughts or significant depression or another mental health problem, I encourage you to seek medical advice to help manage this before considering starting weight-loss injections. For people with milder symptoms, the evidence is more encouraging. A review of research covering more than 107,000 patients found that, compared with placebo, treatment with GLP-1 drugs was not associated with an increased risk of psychiatric adverse events. In fact, treatment was associated with improvements in quality of life (related to improved mental health) and reduced emotional eating.[44]

Liver, kidney and heart disease

As nausea and reduced appetite can reduce fluid intake, some people can become dehydrated when using these

---

44 Pierret A, et al. 'Glucagon-like peptide 1 Receptor agonists and mental health. A systematic review and meta-analysis.' *JAMA Psychiatry*, 2025. doi:10.1001/jamapsychiatry.2025.0679

medications. Vomiting and diarrhoea causes more severe dehydration. Anyone with pre-existing kidney problems could experience worsening of their kidney function from dehydration, and they should be advised to stop taking their weight-loss injections if they experience these side effects.

The manufacturer of Wegovy advises that it should not be used by people with liver disease, as there is limited information on its use in people with severely impaired liver function. It should also be avoided in people with end-stage renal (kidney) failure.

There is an increased risk of metabolic acidosis in people with liver and kidney disease who are taking Mounjaro. This is at least in part due to accumulation of benzyl alcohol, which is an ingredient in the injection solution.

Patients with severe congestive heart failure are advised not to take Wegovy, as it has not been studied in people with this condition.

Gut side effects of Wegovy and Mounjaro

The most common side effects of Wegovy and Mounjaro are related to how they work, and specifically their effect on the gut. Remember that the main effect on the gut is to slow it down. This means that food stays in the stomach for longer, and its passage through the gut takes much longer than normal. If your stomach is full of (old) food, you will not be hungry for a longer period of time. You may also experience burping, possibly with an unpleasant smell and altered taste. Some people experience nausea with a marked loss of appetite, and even vomiting. This in turn can lead to dehydration and undernutrition.

At the other end, the slow passage of food through the gut commonly leads to constipation, bloating or abdominal discomfort. However, some people develop diarrhoea after eating certain foods, especially those high in fat or refined carbohydrates.

These side effects are most marked in the first few days after an injection and generally subside over time. However, they may reappear each time the dose of medication is increased. It is therefore important that you are aware that they might occur, before you start the medication, and that you know how to minimise their impact.

Nausea

Nausea may be severe enough to make you not want to eat or drink at all, therefore it is essential that you drink water to stay hydrated. If you experience vomiting, then sugar-free electrolyte replacements can be very helpful. Fatty foods, spicy foods and refined carbohydrates can make nausea worse, and my advice is to eat small amounts of bland protein-based foods such as chicken breast or even a sugar-free protein shake. Studies have shown that vitamin B6 can help to relieve nausea, and some people find ginger tea or peppermint tea helpful. Prescribed anti-sickness medication may be needed in severe cases.

To repeat, any food you eat will be in your stomach for much longer than is usual, and this can prolong nausea or lead to reflux symptoms. I therefore suggest that you avoid lying down for at least an hour after eating; a gentle walk is a better option as it can aid gut motility and digestion.

Undernutrition

This can be prevented by managing nausea as described above and ensuring you prioritise protein – you should aim for at least 20 grams of protein in every meal.

Constipation

This can also be helped by walking and staying well hydrated. Many of my patients have found that daily psyllium husk (1–2 teaspoons per day, taken in fluid) helps. If you have diabetes, it has also been shown to stabilise glucose levels in some studies.

Diarrhoea

This is usually triggered by certain foods, so it is important to identify these early on. Common culprits include caffeine, fatty foods and high-fibre foods such as certain fruits or vegetables. You may need to limit these. Diarrhoea can also be helped by psyllium husk. It is a good idea to have some over-the-counter loperamide (Imodium) tablets to hand if it becomes difficult to manage. These can be taken for up to five days, but if the diarrhoea persists for longer, it is important to consult your doctor.

The effects of these drugs on the gut can affect other medications you are taking, by reducing the amount of drug that is absorbed. This has been reported with Mounjaro, and it is advised that patients taking warfarin (a blood thinner), digoxin (heart medication) or hormone preparations, including the oral contraceptive pill, should be aware that the effectiveness of these medications could be affected. For this reason, the manufacturers of Mounjaro advise that women on the contraceptive pill also use a barrier method of contraception (such as condoms) for the first month after starting treatment, and after each increase in dose.

Both Wegovy and Mounjaro are prescribed at an initial low dose, and the dose is then increased every four weeks. This allows your body, and especially your gut, to adapt to the effects of the medication, so it is important that you do not increase the dose too quickly. It is also important to **report any side effects to your doctor**. In many cases, I would suggest postponing a dose increase until side effects have settled down. Similarly, if you experience severe side effects after increasing the dose, it is often advisable to return to the lower dose and, if the medication is proving effective on that dose, not to increase the dose again.

Other side effects

Headaches are sometimes experienced when people start treatment. In many cases this results from dehydration, so make sure you drink enough – at least 2 litres per day. It is important to be aware that these drugs can reduce feelings of thirst as well as hunger, and you will likely need to make yourself drink water, rather than relying on feeling thirsty. Fatigue can also result from dehydration, or from the discomfort of the other side effects, particularly in the first few days after an injection.

Hair loss is a quite common effect in anyone who loses a lot of weight, and has been reported by many people taking weight-loss injections. This is not an effect of the medication itself: rather, it is the result of weight loss. It can cause understandable distress, but in almost all cases normal hair growth returns after six months or so.

Psychological problems can be exacerbated by the loss of appetite associated with the injections, because you lose your ability to manage emotions by eating. Comfort or emotional eating is a recognised coping strategy many people employ to help with negative emotions. In some people, this can be an important factor in causing their obesity in the first place. Eating is associated with a release of dopamine in the brain, which has positive effects on mood and is in effect a natural antidepressant. The nausea and loss of appetite caused by weight-loss injections essentially remove this natural antidepressant treatment and can be one reason for the worsening mental health that has been reported in people on GLP-1 injections. Unless alternative support is available, there is a risk that this is enough to lead people to stop the treatment.

Hypotension (low blood pressure) can be associated with dizziness and lethargy. It does not result from the drug itself, but from dehydration that can result from nausea and reduced fluid intake. In many people, weight loss is associated with reducing insulin levels (as part of the reversal of the obesity disease process). Lower insulin has the effect of lowering blood pressure. This is particularly an issue for people who take medication to reduce blood pressure. I generally advise that they monitor their blood pressure at least every week, and if it shows a consistent decline, to discuss with their doctor reducing the dose of any blood pressure medication they are taking.

Allergies such as eczema, other skin rashes or itching have been reported by users of Mounjaro. It contains benzyl alcohol, which may cause allergic reactions.

Hypoglycaemia or low blood glucose levels can occur in people with diabetes who take other diabetes medications, especially insulin or sulfonylurea tablets. If you take medication for diabetes, it is important to discuss this with your doctor before you start taking weight-loss injections, as the dose of your other medications may need to be reduced.

Vitamin deficiencies (such as of vitamin D or B12) often occur in people who are overweight, especially if their diet is high in UPFs of low nutritional value. This has led to the paradox of people who are overfed but undernourished. Reduced food intake can make this problem worse when you are on weight-loss injections, especially if side effects such as vomiting and diarrhoea occur. You can reduce the risk of deficiencies by taking a multivitamin supplement.

Loss of muscle mass while on weight-loss injections has been highlighted in research articles and press reports, and has naturally caused concern. We all lose muscle mass as we get older, and in old age this can lead to sarcopenia (lack of muscle) that is associated with frailty and increased risk of falls. Conventional weight-loss diets lead to loss of some muscle as well as fat. However, in most weight-loss diets, the weight loss is generally much less than occurs with weight-loss injections. In one study, for example, the average weight loss was 6 kg, which is quite a good result from diet changes alone. With injections, however, people are achieving much greater weight loss, and so the overall amount of muscle that could be lost is much greater. Some of the larger trials of Wegovy showed an average weight loss of 16 kg, and up to 40% (6.5 kg) of the weight lost was lean body mass, which includes muscle and bone, rather than fat.[45] Some experts have claimed that this loss of muscle is a result of the body not needing so much muscle because of significant weight loss. This seems to me a spurious unscientific claim. Although the overall body composition has improved (because more fat was lost than lean weight), losing this amount of muscle could cause problems, particularly in older people, in whom muscle mass reduces as part of the ageing process, unless you

---

45 Neeland I, et al. 'Changes in lean body mass with glucagon-like peptide-1-based therapies and mitigation strategies.' *Diabetes Obes. Metab.*, 2024, 26: 16–27.

take steps to maintain it. Drug companies now realise this is a potentially serious issue that needs to be addressed, and are trialling weight-loss drugs taken with muscle-preserving antibodies. Initial results published in June 2025 suggest that such a combination can reduce the loss of lean mass (which includes bone as well as muscle) from 35% to just 7% of weight lost.[46]

The loss of muscle from GLP-1 medications can be exacerbated by the nausea and loss of appetite caused by injections. Muscle loss can be reduced by ensuring a high protein intake while on a weight-reducing diet. This is why I recommend that people ensure they have a good intake of protein at every meal before they start weight-loss injections and while they remain on them.

Age-related macular degeneration is a serious condition that can lead to rapid vision loss in older people. It is not directly related to diabetic eye disease, and risk factors include obesity. A large study from Canada followed up over 100,000 people with Type 2 diabetes. It found that age-related macular degeneration was twice as common (0.2%) in people who had used GLP-1 medications for six months or

---

[46] Regeneron press release. https://investor.regeneron.com/news-releases/news-release-details/results-phase-2-courage-trial-demonstrating-potential-improve

more than in those who had not used the drugs (0.1%). The risk was highest in those who had taken the medication for longer. The researchers suggest that the medications could activate cytokine CXCL12, a chemical involved in immune response that increases levels of vascular endothelial growth factor (VEGF1). This is involved in the development of both diabetic eye disease and age-related macular degeneration.[47]

A rather worrying association has been reported where people using semaglutide had an increased risk of NAION (non-arteritic anterior ischaemic optic neuropathy). This is a rare eye condition, caused by reduced blood flow to the optic nerve. It can lead to sudden loss of vision, and is usually permanent. It normally affects less than 1 in 1000 people but in one study it occurred in over 6% of people taking semaglutide for obesity and in over 8% of people with Type 2 diabetes.[48] This has led to lawsuits being brought against the manufacturer in the USA.

---

[47] Shor R, et al. 'Glucagon-like peptide-1 receptor agonists and risk of neovascular age-related macular degeneration.' *JAMA Ophthalmol.*, 2025, 143: 587–94.

[48] Hathaway J, et al. 'Risk of non-arteritic anterior ischaemic optic neuropathy in patients prescribed semaglutide.' *JAMA Ophthalmology*, 2024, 142: 732–39.

A Guide to Weight Loss Injections

After reading all this, you might decide that these medications are too risky to take. If you have any of the conditions listed in the first part of this chapter, then this is indeed the right option and I would advise that you explore other ways to lose weight. If you do take weight-loss injections, you can expect to experience gut symptoms such as nausea and changes to your bowels as that is, after all, how the drugs work. For some people, these symptoms will be so severe that they cannot continue with the medication. Research suggests that nearly two-thirds of people stop weight-loss injections within a year, and gut effects are a common reason why people stop. Research also shows that many people who stop treatment early begin to regain the weight they have lost.

The next chapter will discuss how you can make injections work best for you.

Chapter 8

How can I maximise the effect, and minimise the side effects, of weight-loss injections?

Stories in the media about weight-loss drugs suggest that they are either amazing wonder drugs that help you to shed pounds with little effort, or they are potentially dangerous medical innovations with nasty side effects that have rightly put people off using them. In the chapters so far, I have tried to provide an objective account of these disparate views. In this chapter we will explore how to find the truth behind these opposing messages, and shape a plan to ensure you can take them safely with the maximum effect and the minimum side effects. Here I would like to emphasise how important it is to view weight-loss injections *as a tool to help you make lifestyle changes*. Let's be clear: all the medical trials of Wegovy and Mounjaro provided support to people to make lifestyle changes while they took the medication. As night follows day, if you take the medication without deliberately trying to make lifestyle changes in addition, then their effect is likely to be less than that seen in the trials. It will also guarantee that you will regain weight when you come off the medication. It's as simple as that.

Here are the steps I recommend. They are designed to maximise the beneficial outcome and to minimise side effects.

Step 1: Set out your goals

For this step, I suggest you buy a notebook where you will document your weight-loss journey, starting off with your goals for using weight-loss injections. You may prefer to use the Notes app on your phone, but I find there is something special about using pen and paper to write down your thoughts. Then make time to sit down and have a good think about why you want to use weight-loss injections. The obvious answer is 'to lose weight', which is a beginning, but you need to follow this up by thinking about the following questions. Write your answers down in your notebook so they will serve as a permanent record of your thoughts and feelings at the start of your journey.

Why do you want to lose weight?

Think about why you want to lose weight. To do this, it might be helpful to let yourself dream about the future – a future where you have already lost weight. How will you feel? How will your life be different? What will you enjoy doing that you currently cannot do? Maybe you used to enjoy a sport or pastime that you have given up all hope of doing again. Or you want to walk upstairs without your knee hurting or getting short of breath. Or you want to be able to get down on the floor to play with your children or grandchildren. There is no right or wrong answer to these questions; what is important is that they help you form a detailed picture of what losing weight will mean for *you*.

How important is it to you that you lose weight?

Are you thinking of using injections because you want to lose weight? Or because others around you are commenting on your weight, perhaps even pressurising you into taking medication? To succeed in losing weight, it must be important to *you*, first and foremost. Yes, others might benefit indirectly if you lose weight, but to put it bluntly, whether you take medication or not is no one else's business – and is certainly not their decision. If it is not really important to you that you lose weight, then it is unlikely that you will put up with having to give yourself an injection every week, especially if you are paying for them yourself. It is also more likely that you will stop using injections at the first sign of any side effects, instead of persevering. By all means, take on board what those close to you are saying when you make your decision to take weight-loss injections. But it must be your decision and no one else's.

Are there any health issues you want to address by losing weight?

Part of your answer to the first question could be related to any health problems you have. I am sure you don't need to be reminded that carrying excess weight can lead to a huge range of health problems, many of which can be reversed by weight loss – and permanently if you succeed in keeping the weight off. To recap what we discussed in Chapter 2, some of the most common problems are listed in Table 8.1.

Table 8.1. Some of the most common health problems associated with being overweight.

Type 2 diabetes	Acid reflux	Gout
Prediabetes	Irregular periods	Migraines
High blood pressure	Erectile dysfunction	Gallstones
High cholesterol level	Low libido	Polycystic ovary syndrome
Arthritis	Depression	Shortness of breath
Back pain	Sleep apnoea	

A Guide to Weight Loss Injections

Maybe you have experienced low mood for many years and assumed this is just how you are. Maybe no one has ever explained to you how losing weight could help this problem, or any of the other problems on the list that you might be experiencing. In my view, modern medicine is all too ready to treat all of these 'symptoms' of obesity with different medications, rather than taking a step back and addressing the underlying cause. After all, as a doctor it is much easier for me to write a prescription (or four) than spend the time with a patient explaining how these problems could be reversed by weight loss and providing them with the necessary support to achieve that. Thankfully things are beginning to change, and the new weight-loss injections make significant weight loss a much more realistic outcome than was previously the case.

How much weight do you want to lose?

This will be partly determined by the reasons for losing weight you have thought about and, possibly, the health problems you want or need to address. In Chapter 2 we discussed BMI, which is a useful but imperfect way of determining if a person is overweight. To recap, if your BMI is 25 or less then this is defined as normal weight, between 25 and 30 is overweight, and above 30 is obesity.

I want to state here that when you lose weight, any weight loss is beneficial, and you certainly do not need to strive for a normal BMI. There are many people who have resolved their health problems through weight loss and are now metabolically healthy but still technically overweight. So, in setting a weight-loss goal it is important to be realistic about how much weight you need to lose to achieve your goal, as well as being realistic about how much you *can* lose. For example, the best results from studies (remember they also included lifestyle advice) showed a weight loss of around 20% body weight. So, if you are about 1.7 m tall (around 5 foot 7 inches) and weigh 110 kg (about 220 pounds or 17 stone), then your BMI will be 38.1. If you do as well as the research trials, you can expect to lose 22 kg at best, down to 88 kg, at which weight your BMI will be 30.4, still within the obese range. The weight loss will greatly benefit your health and could be enough to reverse some weight-related health problems, but you will still be obese. If you need to lose weight to have planned surgery, and the requirement is to achieve a weight loss of 10% or a BMI of less than 35, then this is sufficient to meet that goal. Some people will lose more than that, especially if they adopt the lifestyle changes suggested in Chapter 3; others, if they are unable to tolerate the medication, might lose much less. So, in setting your weight-loss goal, a good starting point is to weigh yourself in pounds or kilos and multiply by 0.8 to see what a realistic best new weight would be. Then ask yourself if your goal is realistic with that new weight. As an example, if one of your goals is to fit into your wedding dress, which fitted you when you were twenty-one, this might not be realistic. But a goal of going down two dress sizes certainly is. And that in itself will be a great achievement.

Do you want the weight loss to be permanent?

The reason I'm asking this question is to get you to really think about what it is that you want to achieve, and how serious you are about achieving it. If your goal is to lose weight for a special occasion, such as a wedding, then you may be motivated to lose weight over a relatively short period of time to achieve that goal. If you are not concerned about your weight afterwards, then it is possible that you will regain the weight you lost – but you will have achieved your goal. If you want to keep the weight off after the event, then you will need to find a way to remain motivated once you have reached your initial goal. Even if your initial goal is a short-term one, I recommend that you start making changes to your diet to plan for long-term changes. And if you are planning long-term changes, it might be helpful to think in terms of what your overall goal is for, say, two years' time, for example, in addition to an initial six-month goal.

I have already mentioned that I am a great believer in committing things to paper. This is not just a personal preference – there is scientific evidence to support this. Research from the Dominican University of California found that people who write down their goals are 42% more likely to reach them than those who don't,[49] so I urge you to set out your goals either below or in a weight-loss diary in your notebook.

My weight-loss goals

I want to lose weight because (give as much detail as possible):

I want to experience these changes in how I feel:

I want to experience these changes to my health:

I want to lose _____ pounds/kilograms in six months.

I want to lose a total of _____ pounds/kilograms by two years.

---

[49] https://www.dominican.edu/sites/default/files/2020-02/gailmatthews-harvard-goals-researchsummary.pdf

Step 2: Set a date and collect data

Having set out your goals, decide on the date you will start your weight-loss journey and commit to making some measurements on that date. On the day, weigh yourself and measure your waist and write these measurements down. If you have health-related goals, such as reversing Type 2 diabetes or reducing your blood pressure, make sure you record relevant measures. You can use a home blood pressure monitor and look up your most recent blood tests for HbA1c (measure of blood glucose) and cholesterol levels. If you have not had them done recently, arrange for a new test to be done before you start your weight-loss journey. When you are thinking about a start date, it is a good idea not to start just before an important occasion or a holiday. Remember, you do not need to have the injections on day one, but when you're planning your start date, schedule an appointment with your GP to see if they can prescribe the medication for you. If not, explore reputable private services to buy the injections. At the time of writing (October 2025) you have a choice of Wegovy or Mounjaro. Mounjaro seems to have the edge in terms of weight loss achieved, but is more expensive. Both are likely to be very effective, compared to any previous treatments you might have tried. Your decision could be based on what is available for your GP to prescribe, the cost of purchasing the medications privately, and any health conditions you have that might make one more suitable than the other (see Chapters 5 and 7).

Give some thought to which day of the week is best for you to take the injections, as they are generally taken on the same day each week. Side effects, if they occur, are more likely in the first few days after an injection. Some people therefore choose to give their injections on Thursdays or Fridays, so they will be at home over the weekend in case they feel unwell.

Write down your plan. You might like to consider the statements listed below.

I will start my weight-loss journey on _____

I will obtain my treatment in time to take my first injection on _____

I will take the injection every _____ each week

On my start date, my measurements are:

Weight:

Waist circumference:

Blood pressure:

Other measurements appropriate to your goals could include:

- for prediabetes or Type 2 diabetes – HbA1c and fasting glucose
- for high cholesterol – total cholesterol, HDL, LDL, triglycerides
- for gout – urate level.

Step 3: Make lifestyle changes before you start injections

The research trials that assessed Wegovy and Mounjaro provided regular support to participants to make changes to their diet and to become more physically active. In the SURMOUNT trial of Mounjaro, for example, this involved contact with a dietitian or other health professional once every two to three weeks throughout the seventy-two weeks of the trial. This does not happen in the real world – unless you are prepared to pay for frequent consultations. I recommend you spend time planning what changes you will make to your diet, and start making those changes *before* you start taking injections. Go back and have a look at the steps I suggested in Chapter 3. Are you ready to start taking one or two of those steps? Remember that fatty foods, spicy foods and refined carbohydrates (such as sugars and starchy foods) can make nausea worse when you start injections. Remember that a good protein intake is vital to help prevent muscle loss, and making changes now to reduce your intake of refined carbohydrates and fatty foods and to increase your protein intake will help make the start of injections less problematic.

Stock up with easy protein-rich foods you enjoy, such as cooked chicken pieces or hard-boiled eggs. Using a protein supplement such as flavoured whey protein powder is a perfectly acceptable way of increasing your protein intake.

Next, have a think about comfort eating or emotional eating. Do you do this? Are there foods or snacks that you eat if you feel stressed, lonely or bored? Weight-loss injections will likely mean you will lose your appetite for them, especially if they are high in sugar. There have been reports of people who have suffered worsening mental health due to being unable to eat their 'comfort foods', as the antidepressant effect of the comfort food is not there. Can you take steps now to try and reduce how much of these foods you eat, perhaps by finding other means of destressing, such as going for a short walk or listening to music?

While I would not encourage you to start a vigorous exercise programme at this stage, making a start with the simple exercises described in Chapter 4 will help maintain muscle mass when you start injections. Going for a short walk after a meal can help you use up some of the energy you have eaten and can greatly help improve mental wellbeing. Can you build these healthy habits into your routine?

Step 4: Review your health and medications

If you have a history of depression or another mental health diagnosis, how are you feeling right now? Weight-loss injections can worsen the symptoms of depression, and it would not be advisable to start taking them if your mental state is affected by depressive symptoms, especially if you have any suicidal thoughts. If you do, it is very important that you seek help from your GP or psychiatric team before starting weight-loss injections. Look again at the section at the start of Chapter 7. Do you have any health conditions that would increase your risk of adverse effects from weight-loss injections? If so, discuss this with your GP, who can advise you whether it would be safe for you to proceed.

In any case, as I have repeatedly advised, see your GP before you start taking injections, especially if you have purchased them yourself; it is essential that your doctor know you are taking the medication in case you develop side effects, and also because some other medications you take may need to be altered. If you take any medications for diabetes, you may need to reduce their dose as weight-loss injections can significantly reduce your glucose level, increasing your risk of hypoglycaemia. Similarly, you may need to reduce the dose of any blood pressure medications once you begin to lose weight. Weight-loss injections can interact with some other medications, such as levothyroxine, fenfluramine (used for some types of seizure) and acenocoumarol (an anticoagulant). Mounjaro can affect the absorption of hormones, including HRT (hormone replacement therapy) and oral contraceptives. Please see your GP to ask their advice about whether you need to make any changes to other medications you are taking.

Step 5: Prepare for your first injection

Both Wegovy and Mounjaro are taken at a low dose to start with but even so, some people find they experience unpleasant side effects straight away. If you have a sensitive gut at the best of times, I would advise you begin on half the normal starting dose (this can easily be done using the injection pens). You might also want to stock up on treatments for common side effects. Table 8.2 shows commonly used preparations that are available without prescription in the UK.

Table 8.2. Some common over-the-counter medications to treat the side effects of weight-loss injections.

Side effect	Treatment
Nausea and vomiting	Cyclizine Cinnarizine (Stugeron) Vitamin B6 (for nausea only)
Diarrhoea	Loperamide (Imodium)
Heartburn/acid reflux	Antacids (e.g. Gaviscon) Esomeprazole (Nexium)
Constipation	Milk of magnesia (treatment) Psyllium husk (prevention)

You may not feel like going out food shopping if you are experiencing side effects, so why not plan ahead for your first week's meals? Remember, you may not be very hungry, so focus on eating protein-rich foods that you enjoy.

Step 6: Start injections

As described in Chapter 5, both Wegovy and Mounjaro are very easy to give yourself, and the injections are generally painless. Make sure you follow the instructions closely and ensure that you give the correct dose. In the UK, each pen contains four doses – so don't inject it all at once! You can take the medication at any time of day. I recommend you decide which time of day works best for you – and when you are least likely to *forget* to take a dose! My suggestion is to give the injection at the start of the day, and to get into the habit of weighing yourself at the same time. But it could be that just before you go to bed, or any other time, works better for you. Stick to that time of day so it builds into your routine, like brushing your teeth. With the medication in your system, your gut will begin to work differently. The most noticeable effect is that you are likely to find you can only manage to eat a fraction of what you could eat previously. As it is important to use the appetite you do have to eat protein, remember to include at least 20 g (and up to 40 g) of protein in each meal, and eat the protein first. As a rough rule of thumb, 100 g of beef, chicken, turkey, tuna and salmon will provide you with 20 g of protein. Three eggs, 200 g Greek yoghurt, cottage cheese and tofu also provide 20 g protein. Lentils or red kidney beans (250 g) do the same, but their high fibre content might not make them a good choice when you are starting off. If the volume of food is too much for you, it is perfectly acceptable to use a protein powder to ensure you get sufficient protein. Your gut will benefit from having some fibre, so try to include some green or salad vegetables if you can. Alternatively, add psyllium husk to yoghurt.

Having less appetite should mean you don't feel like eating snacks between meals. If you do, your slowed-down gut will mean that the snack is still in your stomach when it is time for your next meal, reducing your appetite for that meal. I encourage you not to eat snacks unless you are very hungry – and if you do, make sure it includes protein, such as plain Greek yoghurt or cottage cheese. The need for protein means that I do not recommend skipping meals or prolonged periods of fasting while taking weight-loss injections. Initially, aim for three protein-based meals each day. If you are accustomed to eating late in the evening, aim to bring your last meal forward to no later than 7 p.m. to give your stomach time to empty as much as possible before you go to bed. This will reduce the likelihood of acid reflux or vomiting at night.

Wegovy and Mounjaro reduce thirst as well as appetite for food, so it is important that you remember to drink at least 2 litres of fluids each day. This can include tea and coffee. Some people lose their appetite for alcoholic drinks as well. This will help with weight loss, as alcohol is high in calories. However, if you do drink alcohol, be aware that the medication could make you less tolerant of it – alcohol leads to nausea and dehydration, and so when you are on the injections, your hangovers could be a lot worse. Alcohol also makes some of the gut side effects of the medications worse, so start with one small drink at a time.

Some people tell me that their injections work for a few days and then wear off. By this, they mean that their appetite is severely reduced for two or three days but for the rest of the week it is back to normal. This doesn't mean the drug has stopped working – it just means that the side effects have lessened. The risk is that for the second half of each week, you might revert to eating the foods that made you gain weight in the first place, completely undoing the benefit of the first few days after the injection. But if you retrain your eating habits before starting injections, and make sure you don't have the 'wrong' foods in the house, you can get used to continuing with small protein-based meals until the next injection. The other risk of thinking the medication has stopped working after a few days is that you are tempted to give the next one early, say after five days instead of seven. **You must avoid this at all costs, as it significantly increases the risk of more serious gut side effects.**

Step 7: Record your progress

I believe that record-keeping is an important part of starting any new treatment, so I encourage you to make notes on how you feel each day, what you eat – and, importantly, did any meal cause gut problems afterwards, such as nausea, vomiting or diarrhoea? If so, it's a meal to stay away from for now. I also suggest that you get into the habit of weighing yourself just before you give each injection. The benefit of giving the injection first thing in the morning is that you are weighing yourself when you get up, after going to the toilet but before you have eaten or drunk anything, so it is a true body weight, not influenced by a full bladder or stomach! I recommend you weigh yourself at least every week and write the weight down. Do not expect dramatic changes straight away, but as you start to lose weight, this will become an important record of your progress. It will also help to alert you if your weight loss stalls over a few weeks, and prompt you to review your eating pattern to see if any old habits have crept back in – that is, after all, what habits do. Some people choose to weigh themselves daily. I don't have a problem with that, as long as you are aware that your weight can fluctuate from one day to the next depending on your level of hydration, what you have eaten, whether you have recently opened your bowels, and due to hormonal changes. Some people who have struggled with their weight develop an understandable phobia of weighing scales. If that is the case, then build a habit of weighing yourself every day so it becomes part of your routine, again like brushing your teeth. It can help normalise the process and remove any negative emotions associated with it.

Some people report that they do not see much weight loss initially, but something feels different. That 'something' is that their clothes begin to feel looser, particularly around the waist. This is a really good sign as it indicates you are beginning to lose the excess visceral fat that is so harmful as part of the process causing insulin resistance.

If you do keep these records, then on each 'injection day' I encourage you to look back over the past week – not just to see if you have lost weight and how much, but to look back over the meals you ate, any symptoms you experienced, to consider whether you could do anything differently during the next week to minimise symptoms.

As you come to the end of your first injection pen, or to your fourth injection, weigh yourself and compare that weight with the weight on your first injection day. If you have taken the injection each week, and followed the eating advice I have provided, then it is highly likely that you will have lost weight.

Both Wegovy and Mounjaro recommend increasing the dose each month until you reach the maximum dose. I don't recommend following that advice, since we know that side effects increase with increasing doses and some people do really well losing weight on a lower dose. I recall one patient telling me she needed a higher dose as each injection only 'lasted a few days' – yet over the month she had managed to lose over 6 kg (13 pounds) in weight. I suggested she stay on the same dose and her weight loss continued. So rather than clamouring for a higher dose (with the risk of more side effects) each month, consider whether it would be preferable to stay on the same dose for another month, or longer. If after another month you have not lost any more weight, then you can increase the dose.

Chapter 9

Starting injections – and staying the course

All being well, quite soon after starting treatment with weight-loss injections, you should notice that things are beginning to change. You will probably recognise that you no longer feel hungry like you used to, that your favourite foods seem less appetising, or you have lost the enjoyment you used to take from a glass of wine. All of these are signs that the injections are working. You might also, of course, experience side effects such as nausea or vomiting. Sometimes these side effects are so severe that your only option is to stop taking the injections, for a while at least. While the manufacturer's recommendation is to increase the dose every four weeks, for many people this is unnecessary and it will make any side effects worse. I suggest you only increase the dose if you are not seeing any benefit on your current dose. In Chapter 5, I introduced the concept of microdosing – that is, staying on the lowest dose necessary to help weight loss. Support for this strategy has come from Professor Ben Bikman, a leading authority on metabolic ill health and obesity,[50] and Graham Phillips, a trustee of the Public Health Collaboration, a UK-based charity whose mission is to promote good metabolic health.[51] He is a pharmacist who specialises in the lifestyle management of long-term conditions (he describes himself as 'the pharmacist who gave up drugs'). He advises his patients to start with one injection, and to wait for at least two weeks before considering taking the next dose. This gives them time to properly assess how their body is reacting to the drug, in both good and bad ways, before taking the next injection. Increasingly, I advise my patients to do the same, and it is remarkable how effective this 'microdosing' strategy can be.

Graham has told me that some of his patients have managed to lose weight by only taking one low-dose injection a month. These drugs last a long time in the body and each dose will have an effect for up to twenty days. So, while each injection significantly reduces appetite for the first few days, its effect then wears off gradually, providing an optimal combination of the drug quieting food noise as appetite returns, plus a degree of willpower on the part of the user to stick with their new eating plan until the next injection. This is, it seems

---

50 https://www.washingtontimes.com/news/2025/may/27/microdosing-glp-1-drugs-could-solve-americas-carbohydrate-crisis/
51 https://phcuk.org

to me, a much healthier way of using the injections than moving quickly to a high dose and relying on the injections to remove your appetite completely. A higher dose path not only increases the risk of side effects, but it also increases the risk of you possibly missing out on vital nutrients.

Therefore, when you start your treatment, I encourage you to consider waiting ten to fourteen days between the first few injections. Only reduce the time between injections if you find that you are unable to limit your food intake for that length of time. For the same reasons, do not rush to increase the dose, but only do so when you feel you are no longer benefiting from the medication. Remember, hunger returning between doses is a good thing, as long as you satisfy it by eating meals based on protein and vegetables, and not on sugary snacks. In this way, you are using the medication to help you to change your eating habits, and that will very likely lead to longer-lasting weight loss, even if it is slightly more gradual than when taking higher doses.

The manufacturer states that Wegovy pens, which contain four doses, should be used within six weeks, so extending the time between injections should enable you to comply with this timeframe. Interestingly, however, Ozempic pens are said to be useable for up to eight weeks. I can see no logical reason for this difference (apart from encouraging you to use the doses sooner), and Wegovy is also likely to be effective for up to eight weeks, especially if it's kept in the refrigerator. The manufacturer of Mounjaro, by contrast, states that the pens should be used within thirty days, which means if you extend the time between injections, you will breach this limit. Therefore, using Mounjaro limits the scope to extend the interval between injections. Having said that, I have had patients who have done this without any problem, although I advise all patients to keep the pen in the refrigerator, to minimise the risk of degradation of the active ingredient.

Side effects can occur, even at lower doses, especially when you start treatment or move to a higher dose. Some of the gut side effects are made worse by certain foods, such as fatty foods, sugary foods, or excessive fibre (for example, a large portion of vegetables or salad). In Chapter 8, I emphasised the importance of keeping records and monitoring your progress. As part of this, I encourage you to keep a diary of what you eat (just a few brief details), your feelings and any symptoms you experience – good or bad. This will help you identify how you respond to each dose and help you to decide when to take the next dose. Remember that these drugs work by changing how your gut works, and so some changes such as bloating, heartburn, constipation and diarrhoea are very likely. If they are mild and/or temporary, there is no need to stop the injections. Make sure you have the remedies recommended in Chapter 7 to help you manage if they arise.

A Guide to Weight Loss Injections

An example of your diary might look like this.

Date	weight	dose	how do I feel today?	food noise	cravings	hunger	nausea	vomiting	diarrhoea	headache
1	120kg	0.25mg	good	low	low	low	none	no	no	no
2			ok	no	no	no	mild	no	no	mild
3			awful	no	no	no	bad	once	no	bad
4			nauseated	no	no	no	moderate	no	a bit	quite bad
5			ok	no	no	no	mild	no	no	no
6			ok	no	no	a bit	no	no	no	no
7				no	no	a bit	no	no	no	no
8	118kg		good	no	no	a bit	no	no	a bit	no
9										
10										

This shows that symptoms were at their worst two days after the injection, but quickly improved. It also shows that after seven days there was no food noise or cravings and very little hunger, so the patient could safely delay their next injection for a few more days at least. Increasing hunger over the next few days isn't a reason to rush to the next dose, unless it is associated with troublesome food noise or cravings. Keeping a food diary alongside this checklist will help you identify any foods that are associated with particularly unpleasant symptoms and will enable you to create a list of foods to avoid, especially in the early stages. Remember to drink, as your thirst might be also reduced. It is also a good idea to record your fluid intake.

From all the above, it follows that there is no need to increase the dose if you are in control of your food intake and you are losing weight. The time to consider increasing the dose is when you are injecting every seven days and finding that you are struggling to control your food intake because of hunger, food cravings or food noise. Then you can move to the next dose and start the process again, monitoring the effect of each injection and – ideally – again being able to wait ten to fourteen days before the next one. If at any stage you develop more severe side effects, manage them as advised in Chapter 7 and delay your next dose until they have resolved. If you have felt particularly bad, I recommend that you consider not only delaying but also reducing the dose to the next dose down. If you then feel in a position to do so, you can increase the dose after a few weeks. But if you experience a bad reaction a second time, it likely means that this dose is simply too high for you and you will need to remain on the lower dose for the remainder of your treatment. You are still likely to benefit from the lower dose, and you are more likely to reach your weight-loss goal by staying on medication than stopping it prematurely, especially if you are still experiencing food cravings.

If you find that you cannot tolerate the lowest dose, then it is definitely worth switching to a different drug. I have had some patients who have had very bad reactions to Wegovy and then switched to Mounjaro and experienced no problems at all thereafter (and vice versa).

If you are unfortunate enough to experience a severe side effect such as pancreatitis (see below), gallstones, or to develop medullary thyroid cancer (which is extremely rare), it is not advisable for you to restart medication.

This strategy should help you achieve your weight-loss goals and discover a new way of eating while on treatment. In Chapter 11 we will discuss when and how to come off treatment. Meanwhile, life carries on for the time that you are taking injections. The next section of this chapter guides you through some of the things that might happen when you are on treatment.

Illness

If you become unwell while on treatment, my advice is to wait until you are better before taking your next injection. This is because very occasionally, serious illness, such as pancreatitis, can be a side effect of the medication. The signs of pancreatitis are severe upper abdominal pain, along with nausea and vomiting, and often accompanied by a fever. If you develop these symptoms, seek medical advice urgently. Any illness that causes vomiting or diarrhoea risks you becoming dehydrated – clearly, weight-loss injections can make these symptoms worse so are best avoided until you have recovered. Other illnesses that do not cause gut symptoms, especially those associated with a high temperature, can also cause dehydration, and so the safest strategy is to wait until you are better before taking your next injection. If you have stopped treatment for more than two weeks then it may be advisable to restart at a lower dose as otherwise you may experience more marked side effects. Please seek advice from your prescribing doctor.

Surgery

As weight-loss injections slow down the actions of the gut, food can stay in the stomach for much longer than is normal. There have been cases where this has caused problems with vomiting after anaesthesia. In 2023, the American Society of Anaesthesiologists recommended pausing injections for at least a week before surgery. In contrast, a consensus statement from UK specialists in 2025 suggests there is no need to do this.[52] These medications are still relatively new and so, given the specialists' differing opinions, I recommend that if you are having planned surgery, it is vital that you inform the surgical team that you are taking weight-loss injections as, in certain situations, it may be advised you should omit a dose.

---

52 El-Boghdadly K, et al. 'Elective peri-operative management of adults taking glucagon-like peptide-1 receptor agonists, glucose-dependent insulinotropic peptide agonists and sodium-glucose cotransporter-2 inhibitors: A multidisciplinary consensus statement.' *Anaesthesia*, 2025, 80:412–24.

Pregnancy

Studies in animals suggest there is a higher risk of miscarriage and congenital abnormalities associated with the drugs, so women of childbearing age are recommended to avoid getting pregnant while on treatment, and to use additional barrier methods of contraception (e.g. condoms) as the injections can affect the effectiveness of the contraceptive pill. This is essential even for women who consider themselves infertile because they have not previously been able to conceive. One of the beneficial effects of weight loss is to restore hormonal cycles that have been disrupted due to insulin resistance associated with obesity. The net result is that the treatment can increase fertility, and thus the chances of pregnancy occurring. It is not so surprising, then, that women have become pregnant while on weight-loss injections, and many have gone on to deliver healthy babies. If you do become pregnant, it is essential to stop taking the injections and seek medical advice.

Special occasions

Special occasions that involve food (think birthdays, barbecues or bank holiday get-togethers) are often a challenge for people trying to lose weight, and always have been, especially if the food on offer is precisely the sort you are trying to avoid.

The added complication of weight-loss injections is you will probably have very little appetite or feel too nauseated to eat anything. You may therefore wish to adjust the timing of an injection by a few days so you can enjoy a special occasion and maybe eat more than you normally would. However, I would advise against throwing all caution to the wind by reverting to your previous eating habits, as this could lead to a significant setback in your weight-loss journey, especially if you eat foods that lead to the return of food cravings. If you feel there is a risk of that, my advice is not to deviate from your new eating pattern. If the occasion involves a meal at a restaurant, hopefully you will be able to choose a suitable dish on the menu and in not too large a portion, so it doesn't aggravate any gut issues. Some people choose to eat a starter instead of a main. A buffet will allow you to choose exactly what you put on your plate, but a sit-down function such as a wedding could be more of a challenge, as you will obviously have less control over what is put in front of you. In that situation I would encourage you to be explicit by politely declining a main course and/or dessert. Try to avoid the trap of (entirely naturally) feeling you *ought* to eat all the food that you are given. Some people find this hard to do, especially if they were told in childhood that they had to clear their plate at every meal.

Telling others

It is essential that you tell your GP and any other health professionals who are advising you on your health that you are taking weight-loss injections. As we can see from every newspaper, magazine, Instagram reel, TikTok post and breakfast TV programme, a host of celebrities and influencers seem to be very happy to share their experiences – the good, the bad and the awful – of taking the injections. But most of us may wish to be more private about our health; many people who live with obesity have experienced judgemental attitudes and stigma that have led them to feel a sense of shame about their weight. However, I encourage you to find the words to tell family members and friends that you have opted for the injections, so they understand why your eating habits have changed, why you may be feeling less well than usual, or why you may not feel up to eating out or drinking like you used to. But choose your words carefully. Rather than saying 'I am taking weight-loss jabs', you could say something like 'I am following a weight management programme that includes medications and a change in my diet.' You could follow this with 'So please don't offer me sugary foods/biscuits/snacks as I am choosing not to eat them at the moment!' Or 'I am choosing smaller meals at the moment' or 'I am choosing not to drink alcohol'. This way, you are letting people know that you are taking a medication, but the focus is on the dietary changes you are making and that *you* are taking the lead in choosing to make those changes.

You can use similar phrases, though without mentioning medication, when eating out. At most restaurants now, the server will ask if you have any allergies or dietary requirements, and this is a golden opportunity to ask if they can recommend a smaller dish that is not spicy, or whatever your requirement is.

Holidays

A few years ago, I spent time professionally in Bermuda, where I helped to set up a lifestyle programme to help people reverse Type 2 diabetes. This was before the widespread use of weight-loss injections, and required people to use their willpower to reduce their intake of sugary and starchy foods. As is the case on many small islands that rely on imported food, fresh, healthy foods are relatively expensive in Bermuda, so UPFs from the USA make up a high proportion of residents' overall calories. As a result, there is a very high rate of obesity on the island – and a whole industry dedicated to various weight-loss programmes.

At least some of these included what people referred to as a 'cheat day', often a Saturday or Sunday, and I was often asked about such cheat days. It occurred to me that if this means going wild for one day every week, then this could easily undo all the good done by following a healthy eating plan during the rest of the week. My advice was to by all means enjoy an *occasional* treat day – perhaps a day where you enjoy a non-food-related treat to mark a special occasion or achievement, such as meeting a weight-loss goal – but not a cheat day, and certainly not every week. From a commercial point of view, I can see the benefit to people who run weight-loss programmes to encourage cheat days, as it will prolong the time that people remain their paying customers! But from a weight-loss point of view – especially from a behaviour-change point of view – it really makes no sense at all.

I do not see the same focus on cheat days in the UK, but I often see how holidays can undo months of weight-loss progress. In my experience, two types of holiday seem particularly problematic: cruises and trips to the USA. Both involve being exposed to huge amounts of unhealthy foods. Sure, you can seek out healthy options, but often the ready availability of unhealthy foods seems to take precedence. I therefore strongly recommend that people do not miss a dose before a holiday so that they can enjoy the food on offer – even if it is to celebrate a special occasion. It is really so easy to pile the pounds back on in a very short time. Look, if the idea of going on a cruise with a limited appetite (so you are unable to eat much of the food on offer) has not much appeal, then perhaps a cruise is not the best type of holiday to choose.

Changing other medications

Since many health problems are related to obesity, or at least made worse by it, so also are many health problems improved by losing weight. If you are on treatment for diabetes or high blood pressure, it is important that you keep an eye on your glucose and blood pressure levels. As you take weight-loss injections, you will likely find that as you lose weight, your glucose levels and blood pressure come down. This often means that your dose of medications for diabetes and blood pressure need to be reduced – and possibly stopped altogether. Failure to do this could result in low blood pressure or dangerously low blood glucose levels, especially if you are taking insulin or a sulfonylurea tablet (such as gliclazide or glimepiride). There may be other medications, such as levothyroxine (taken for an underactive thyroid gland), that could be affected in a similar way.

This is another reason why it is essential that you tell your GP or other regular prescriber (such as your pharmacist) that you are taking weight-loss injections. They will advise you how to check if you need to reduce any other medications. Other conditions that can be improved by weight loss include oesophageal reflux (which causes heartburn), gout, poor sleep, arthritis and back pain – and you may be able to stop medications for these problems as well. Wouldn't that be great?

Chapter 10

The importance of managing stress, mood and sleep while on weight-loss injections

Stress: the modern scourge

Many of us live in a state of stress. While we might not feel obviously stressed, the way we live nowadays can lead to a constant state of low-level stress that is harmful to our health. Thirty years ago, for most people work started and finished when they arrived and left the workplace. Period. Today, when we can access our email and texts on our mobile phones, we are at risk of being always available. We also take our work home with us, and even to bed with us.

To mobile phones, TikTok, Instagram and email we can add the impact of computer games and 24/7 TV, including a news cycle that never switches off, internet shopping and banking, and Netflix's and its competitors' bingeable series, accompanied by the inevitable ads to keep us watching and coming back for more. These all have the potential to raise stress levels, to disturb our sleep or both. Remember, none of these things existed thirty years ago...

In many respects, these advances in technology and media have been enjoyable and beneficial. We no longer have to wonder where anyone is, as almost everyone now has a personal tracking device, also known as a mobile phone. Yet over these thirty years, as well as seeing increasing rates of obesity, we have also seen increases in a whole host of other conditions, including Type 2 diabetes, depression, mood disturbances and chronic fatigue. So, is modern living that bad for us?

In a word – yes. For previous generations, their lifestyle was dictated by geography and daylight. Without the means to move quickly around, people stayed in relatively close-knit communities and lived and worked close to where they grew up. The world was largely rural and work was necessarily within walking distance. Once it got dark, it was time to switch off the brain and go to sleep – or to stay up in rather dim candlelight. Life wasn't always easy, but it was much closer to the sort of living for which our bodies evolved.

Many of the body's processes are controlled by hormones, which vary according to what is called a circadian rhythm. This means that the hormone levels in the bloodstream change over each twenty-four-hour period. One of the key hormones is cortisol, the body's natural steroid. Its levels rise during the early morning, to ensure that we are wide awake and alert at the start of the day and to prepare us for the day ahead. Then, as the day progresses, our cortisol levels naturally decline. They reach their lowest levels late at night, to enable the body to sleep.

Cortisol is the body's main stress hormone, and is increased whenever we are under any kind of stress. The actions of cortisol are to increase blood glucose levels and to ratchet up the immune system as part of what is called the fight-or-flight response, to enable us to fight or run away from an enemy, and to help the body heal following any physical injury. These are all good things if we are in serious trouble, such as being attacked by a wild animal. In that situation, our cortisol level increases to help us survive the attack, then naturally lowers to normal levels.

The trouble is, our body's hormones cannot readily distinguish between that type of emergency and the multitude of stresses that impact upon our modern lives. As a result, any emotional, physical or mental stress can cause our cortisol level to spike. It could be because of a serious illness, job or money worries, or living in an unhappy relationship. It could also be because we are rushing around doing one job after another, because we are stuck in traffic and late for an appointment, or because we have been unfriended on Facebook. The net effect is that all too often our cortisol level is high, meaning our immune system is constantly primed and our energy stores mobilised to cause blood glucose – and also insulin levels – levels to rise. If your cortisol levels are constantly raised, the accompanying high insulin levels drive hunger and weight gain, sabotaging your attempts to lose weight and reverse the obesity disease process. It stands to reason. Indeed, many people with diabetes find that when they are in a stressful situation, their blood glucose levels can go very high indeed – even if they are following a healthy diet. To summarise: effectively managing your stress is essential, not only for your mental wellbeing, but as an important step in improving metabolic health and losing weight.

Just as we must learn how to undo the harmful effect of the unhealthy food that surrounds us, so too – if we really want to maximise our health – must we learn how to undo the harmful effects of our always-on lifestyles. So how can we do that? There are a number of things that will help. Some will apply to you; others will not. One that I think is universally relevant is the need to take breaks during the day. For much of my working life in a busy hospital, I would work for up to ten hours without stopping. I would grab a coffee during the clinic and take it back to my consultation room and I would munch on a sandwich while checking emails at lunchtime. Very often I would spend the entire day in one room. It became normal, and I would get home exhausted and not very nice to be with.

Now the irony is that the hospital was on a very pleasant greenfield site, with an inviting duck pond in the middle. On occasions when I was feeling very stressed, I would buy a couple of chocolate bars and go out to walk around the pond – I quickly discovered it had a noticeably calming effect. Now I realise it would have been much better if I had built such breaks into my daily routine. Had I done so, I probably wouldn't have needed the 'comforting' chocolate bars.

In 2013, I moved to Belgium and worked in an office environment. Like the French, the Belgians value their lunch hour, and every day, work paused for an hour in the middle of the day. While I didn't want to spend the whole time eating, I often took the opportunity to take a walk in the forest across the road. I came back relaxed and refreshed and I am sure that my afternoon productivity benefited as a result. Indeed, during that period, I attended a seminar where we were shown brain activity scans of a person, taken after they had been sitting down for two hours, and after a twenty-minute walk. The difference was incredible. After sitting down, large parts of the brain had shut off – gone into 'sleep mode', yet after a short walk, the brain was all lit up and firing on all cylinders.

I now make it a habit to get some fresh air every morning. I am lucky enough to live near the coast, so I can walk out with my dog and be on the clifftop in just a few minutes. If I am at work, then I make a point of leaving the building and going out to buy a cup of coffee. Unless it is pouring with rain, I sit outside for a few minutes just enjoying being, before returning to my clinic. Just a short break outside can not only wake up the brain (thereby using up more energy, so less is stored as fat), but it also helps to disrupt stress, helping reduce cortisol levels – and bringing all the benefits that come with that.

The link between obesity and mental wellbeing

In addition to the stresses that we all experience as part of modern life, obesity is also linked to various mental health conditions, including depression, anxiety, low self-esteem and social isolation. The relationship is bidirectional, meaning obesity can contribute to mental health problems, and mental health conditions can also lead to weight gain. Furthermore, weight stigma and bias can negatively impact mental wellbeing.

The relationship between obesity and mental health is complex and not fully understood. However, it is clear that obesity can worsen existing mental health conditions and that mental health problems (and many medications used to treat them) can contribute to weight gain.

Apart from distress directly arising from living with obesity, there is a strong link between depression and obesity, with evidence that insulin resistance (as occurs in most cases of obesity) can affect the chemical balance in the brain and increase the likelihood of symptoms of depression. One study found that adults with obesity had a 55% higher risk of developing depression, and those with depression had a 58% increased risk of obesity.[53] Unfortunately, we often use sweet foods as a pick-me-up if we are feeling down, stressed or just want to cheer ourselves up. Not only will this worsen obesity and increase the risk of developing diabetes, but sugar has a direct effect on the brain and causes a feeling of wellbeing. Some people call it a sugar rush. Others describe getting sugar cravings – and as the effect wears off, they are prompted to eat yet more. A vicious cycle then sets in motion, where a person with insulin resistance is more liable

---

53 Jakela M, 'Obesity as a causal risk factor for depression: Systematic review and meta-analysis of Mendelian randomization studies and implications for population mental health.' *J. Psychiatr. Res.*, 2023, 163: 86–92.

to feeling depressed. They may then resort to eating sugary foods to improve their mood (which it does in the very short term), but that also worsens their insulin resistance, which can lead to even lower mood, more sugar intake and so on. And as we know, as well as affecting mood, insulin resistance also increases body weight, blood glucose levels, and the risk of developing Type 2 diabetes.

There is also evidence that eating processed foods is associated with an increased risk of depression and mild cognitive impairment. So, not only do sugar and other processed foods increase the risk of metabolic ill health and obesity, they also increase the risk of depression. There is, therefore, evidence of a circular causal link between an unhealthy diet and poor mental health. Poor mental health can lead to unhealthy eating, and an unhealthy diet can contribute to poor mental health. We also know that poor mental health can be associated with other unhealthy behaviours, such as being physically inactive.

Similarly, people with bipolar disorder may use food to cope with their condition, leading to weight gain. While there is no direct evidence that obesity causes bipolar disorder, there is exciting evidence coming out about how bipolar disorder and other mental health conditions can be effectively managed by making changes to your diet and losing weight, lending support to the hypothesis that the current high prevalence of mental health disorders is related to modern lifestyle and diet.[54]

Obesity, and trying to manage it, can also be associated with anxiety disorders. The stress of managing weight, social stigma and potential health complications can all contribute to anxiety. Negative body image and poor self-esteem are common among individuals with obesity, often stemming from societal pressures and weight stigma. These in turn can lead to social isolation, rejection by peers, and difficulties in relationships.

Minimising stress and maximising mental health

It is unsurprising that people living with obesity and whose diet is not nutritious can experience higher levels of stress and depression. While that sounds pretty depressing, the good news is that a healthier diet can improve mental health. A healthy diet of fresh, unprocessed foods, avoiding sugars and refined carbohydrates, will help reduce insulin resistance and inflammation, improving both physical and mental health.

Physical activity can also improve our mood. I hope I have already made the case for one of the quickest (and cheapest)

---

54 Campbell IH, et al. 'A pilot study of a ketogenic diet in bipolar disorder: Clinical, metabolic and magnetic resonance spectroscopy findings.' *BJPsych Open*, 2025, 11(2): e34.

win-wins: people, go out for a walk! A short walk can make us feel better – more alert and happier. A few years ago, some very interesting research was published that showed that spending two hours a week in nature is associated with better health and wellbeing. In that study, nature didn't mean being in open countryside; it also included a walk in a town park, or along a riverbank.[55] The two hours didn't need to be taken in one go, but could be made up of several smaller periods, such as fifteen-minute breaks each day, perhaps with a longer walk at weekends. This effect wasn't just due to the increased physical activity, as it was also seen in people with disabilities. There is something calming about being surrounded by nature.

More intensive exercise – such as running, cycling or swimming – increases the production of endorphins. These are released by the hypothalamus in response to pain or stress, and have the effect of relieving pain and creating a general feeling of wellbeing. Have a think about what changes you can build into your daily routine that could reduce feelings of being constantly under stress. We cannot necessarily avoid the situations that cause us to become stressed, but we can learn to be more aware of how stress makes us feel or behave.

---

55 White MP, et al. 'Spending at least 120 minutes a week in nature is associated with good health and wellbeing.' *Scientific Reports*, 2019, 9: article 7730.

If you can recognise the symptoms, then you should be able to take corrective action to reduce the effect of stress on your body.

From the previous chapters, it should be evident that while a diagnosis of clinical obesity can be associated with serious health problems, there are huge numbers of things you can do to prevent those problems happening and to improve your health now and in the future. However, it will require you to make permanent changes to what you eat, and possibly to other aspects of your daily life. While these changes will bring benefits, change can create its own challenges or bumps along the road. Being overweight or obese can also have impacts on your psychological health. Any change can be stressful, so making lifestyle changes to help reverse obesity can, in the short term at least, make your mental health worse before it gets better. It is also important to acknowledge the mental health impact of using injections to manage weight.

For many people who use these medications for obesity, it is the first time they have had to put a needle into themselves. Most people find the needles painless, and after a bit of understandable apprehension, soon have no difficulty in injecting themselves. However, merely the thought of an injection can cause anxiety in some people, especially if they have had painful experiences in the past. Some people have a genuine needle phobia, which no amount of reassurance about the tiny size of the needles and painless nature of injections can overcome. In either situation, the stress caused by anxiety about injections can potentially cancel out their benefit.

If you have anxieties about self-injection, please seek advice on addressing these before embarking on treatment, so you can maximise the benefit you get from the injections. It could be as simple as asking someone else to administer the first few injections for you, or you might need more in-depth counselling. If you really cannot face the idea of injections, maybe it would be best to wait a year or two until the new tablet forms of these drugs, such as Orforglipron, become available (see Chapter 13).

If you are having treatment for a psychiatric disorder, I reiterate my advice in Chapter 7: please seek medical advice before starting weight-loss injections, as there have been reports that they can make symptoms worse. In Chapter 7, we also discussed how loss of appetite with weight-loss treatments can worsen symptoms of anxiety and depression, as emotional or comfort eating will be more difficult and could potentially make you feel sick. This emphasises the benefits of making changes to your diet before you start injections.

A Guide to Weight Loss Injections

Looking after you

In a busy world, where many of us must juggle work and family responsibilities, it can be easy to forget to look after ourselves. Yet, if you are obese and want to lose weight, it is essential that you take the time to prioritise your own health. So far, we have largely focused on improving physical health. But it is also important to look after our own mental wellbeing. We all need some 'me time' – a regular time out just for us. But many of us are not very good at doing this.

I have seen many patients over the years who prioritise the needs of their children, spouse or elderly parents over their own needs. That can lead them to become drained and exhausted and in a constant state of stress. But if you have a health condition that requires your attention, not attending to your own needs can be positively harmful to you. Looking after yourself is not being selfish. After all, if we don't value ourselves enough to look after ourselves and cater for our needs, then who will? And if, as a result, something happens to us, then those who are dependent on us will be left to fend for themselves. So is there something that you would like to do, just for you, once or twice a week? It could be anything: an exercise class, learning a new skill, learning to play an instrument or even taking the time to sit down and watch your favourite TV programme. The two things that matter are that it's something that gives you pleasure and it does not involve eating unhealthy food.

Sleep

The ultimate rest is, of course, sleep, and allowing ourselves to get a good night's sleep is so important. All too often, however, we squeeze sleep in only when we have finished our day's business, regardless of when that is. I mentioned that a few years ago I lived in Belgium, and there I worked in an international policy role that meant I was in contact with people from all around the world in every time zone. Consequently, emails would come in thick and fast around the clock – right to my phone. Recognising that this could disrupt my relaxation and sleep, I had to plan times, such as in the evenings and overnight, when I'd leave my phone on my desk, well away from the bedroom. Today's phones have a 'do not disturb' facility to turn off notifications.

Undoubtedly, having access to friends and work colleagues at all times does have its benefits. But it also has its downsides. What might be the effect of receiving a work email as you are going to bed? Or a non-urgent but difficult text from a family member, moments before you are about to set off for a nice evening out – or even worse, while you are out? At best, they will cause a certain amount of stress. At worst, they will make you feel that you have to change your plans or stay up to deal with it. Or you might lie awake at night worrying about it. Some employers are now beginning to acknowledge this as a problem, and more enlightened companies are starting to issue policy bans on using work email outside normal working hours. They recognise that employees will be far more productive during the day after a good night's sleep than if they are up at all hours responding to 'urgent' emails. However, recent research shows that such companies are in a minority. In Germany, it is common for companies to actively discourage employees from working outside normal work hours, and in 2021 Portugal introduced a 'right to disconnect' law that bans employers from contacting employees outside working hours. The current UK government is considering non-binding guidance for employers to respect a right to disconnect, similar to the situation in Belgium and Ireland.[56]

Social media – and other modern technology – is just one cause of disturbed sleep. Some of us work in a culture where it is considered 'virtuous' to stay up until 3 a.m. working to meet a deadline. How wrong we are. It has been shown that poor sleep has a bigger impact on driving performance than drinking alcohol. A few years ago I had to drive home from

---

56 https://theweek.com/politics/banning-emails-after-5pm-what-the-uk-can-learn-from-portugals-right-to-disconnect-rule

the airport after an overnight transatlantic flight, where I had less than two hours' poor-quality sleep. The drive took about two hours, and I was aware that my reaction times were slowed and it was a real struggle to stay awake. Halfway home, I felt in desperate need of coffee and sugar to keep me alert. This wasn't just psychological. Poor sleep leads to increased levels of – you guessed it – cortisol, which increases appetite but decreases satiety, so even after you eat more, you still feel hungry. You will not be surprised to learn that, even in people without diabetes, blood sugar levels are higher after disturbed sleep, setting off the train of insulin resistance, increased fat storage and weight gain. Good sleep, on the other hand, has the opposite effect – it is incredibly beneficial.

In his book *The 4 Pillar Plan*, Dr Rangan Chatterjee includes a whole chapter on how to improve sleep, with many helpful tips. These include having screen-free time for ninety minutes before going to bed.[57] Quite apart from the impact that stress from emails and social media messages can have on disturbing sleep, the blue light emitted by screens tricks our brains into thinking it is still daytime, disturbing the hormone changes that make us sleepy and risking keeping us awake into the night – a double whammy. Instead, try

---

[57] Chatterjee R (2017), *The 4 Pillar Plan: How to relax, eat, move and sleep your way to a longer, healthier life*. Penguin.

A Guide to Weight Loss Injections

relaxing and aiming (where possible) to avoid mental stress in the late evening, have a period of phone-free time before bed, and sleep in absolute darkness.

Chapter 11
Successfully coming off injections

Throughout this book I have tried to emphasise that weight-loss injections should be seen as a medium-term support to help you lose weight while changing your relationship with food by taking away food noise and food cravings. And while some experts feel that these drugs should be used as a long-term treatment, like blood pressure medications, for example, there are significant side effects associated with weight-loss injections, and limited knowledge about adverse effects of long-term treatment.

Bizarre as it may seem, I recommend that you begin to plan for how you will stop treatment before you even start the injections. It is why I suggest making changes to your diet before you start injections, as you will need to continue your new eating pattern afterwards, and the earlier you start, the more likely it is that you will maintain those changes in the long term.

In Chapter 8 we talked about the importance of identifying your goals from treatments, and thinking about what you hope to achieve. All the large studies using weight-loss injections suggest that significant weight loss occurs during the first eighteen months of treatment, so realistically treatment should not need to continue beyond two years. So as you approach the point of reaching your weight-loss goal, you should consciously and actively ensure you have put everything in place that will enable you to come off the medication successfully without regaining weight. In this chapter I will explain the steps that can help you achieve that.

In reality, despite their best intentions, many people stop the medications without reaching their weight-loss goal. Some studies describe real-world data on drug usage by people who are using the injections as a treatment for a condition rather than as a clinical trial. Real-world data generally shows drugs to be less effective than in a clinical trial, as during a trial the people taking the drugs receive regular monitoring and support and are by definition motivated to take part in the trial, as it is voluntary. An analysis of real-world data from a large number of patients in the USA shows that around 65% of people stop weight-loss injections within the first year. One of the biggest reasons for stopping is because of the gut side effects. Other reasons include the high cost of the injections, especially among the people who are paying for them themselves.[58]

Another reason for stopping injections is due to drug shortages. In the years since the COVID pandemic, there have been reported shortages of many medications – something that is much more common now than previously. And this includes shortages of GLP-1 medications, because the demand has far exceeded the supply. On current trends, that demand is going to increase significantly, and it is quite possible that there will be shortages again in the future. At worst, a sudden unavailability of the injections could lead you to go back to your previous eating patterns and to regain the weight you had succeeding in losing. It's another good reason to have a well-thought-out plan for how you will manage life after injections – and a plan you can put into place at very short notice, if needed.

Finally, it is important to understand that in the UK Wegovy is currently limited to two years of treatment. Patients using these injections are going to have to plan for when they come off them.

---

[58] Rodriguez PJ, et al. 'Discontinuation and reinitiation of dual-labeled GLP-1 receptor agonists among US adults with overweight or obesity.' *JAMA Netw. Open.*, 2025, 8(1): e2457349.

Just as I recommend that these drugs are started at a very low dose that is increased very slowly and only when necessary, I recommend the same approach when stopping the medication.

Many people stop taking WLIs when they experience side effects, but if you do this, you risk regaining the weight you have lost. So rather than stopping completely in the event of side effects, I recommend that you reduce the dose and/or increase the time between doses from seven to ten days or longer. That should reduce side effects while your body is still benefiting from having the medication. If you are paying for the injections yourself, using a lower dose or a longer interval will reduce the cost and perhaps make it more feasible for you to continue until you have reached your weight-loss goal.

Most of the drug trials funded by the manufacturers of these medications show that, once people have stopped taking them, the weight piles back on. As an example, in the STEP 1 study of Wegovy, the 15% weight loss at one year had reduced to just 6% after a year without injections, and was potentially back at square one before two years. And the risk is that most of the regained weight is likely to be fat, rather than muscle, so that you end up back at your starting weight but with less muscle to help support you and get you around.

It is easy to see why the manufacturers wish to convey this message, as it lends support to the idea that people with obesity need to take these injections over the long term, as that will help their profits. However, several studies coming out of the USA have shown that it is possible to maintain weight loss after coming off injections. One study looked at the effect of using older weight-loss medications to help keep weight off after stopping injections. In this study, around 80% of people used metformin and were able to maintain their weight loss. Metformin is a commonly used medication for Type 2 diabetes which can have an effect in reducing appetite – but in the UK it is not licensed for people who do not have Type 2 diabetes. Other medications used in that study included phentermine (an appetite suppressant that is a controlled drug and so not widely available in the UK), topiramate (used for epilepsy and not licensed for weight loss in the UK) and bupropion.[59] This is the drug in Zyban, used to help people stop smoking. It is also one of the active ingredients in Mysimba, which is licensed in the UK for weight loss, but not available on the NHS. It works by reducing food cravings and could be an option for people who experience a return of food cravings as they reduce their dose of Wegovy or Mounjaro.

---

[59] Paddu NU, et al. 'Weight maintenance on cost-effective anti-obesity medications after 1 year of GLP-1 receptor agonist therapy: A real world study.' *Obesity (Silver Spring)*, 2024, 32(12): 2255–63.

Virta Health is a US-based organisation that supports people to lose weight and reverse Type 2 diabetes and other weight-related health problems. They encourage patients to follow a very low carbohydrate diet, and have found that this enables many people to come off weight-loss injections without regaining weight. Many of these were people with Type 2 diabetes, and they often continued taking metformin and potentially benefited from its effect in reducing appetite.[60] But these findings do suggest that if you follow my low-carbohydrate, high-protein dietary plan in Chapter 3 then there is a good chance that you will be able to come off your injections without regaining weight.

Remember that your body produces GLP-1 naturally, and you can use your diet to maximise its own production. The foods that will most help include protein, especially eggs, fibre (in vegetables, lentils and nuts) and olive oil. As discussed in Chapter 3, I recommend that you include these in your diet before you start injections, and especially before you begin to come off them. Everyone is different, with different reasons for coming off the injections at different times, and so we cannot cover every eventuality here. Even so, the

---

60 McKenzie A, et al. 'Impact of glucagon-like peptide-1 agonist deprescription in Type 2 diabetes in a real-world setting: A propensity score matched cohort study.' *Diabetes Ther.*, 2024, 15: 843–53.

following steps are designed to guide you through the process of coming off your weight-loss injections.

Step 1: Plan ahead

In Chapter 7, I encouraged you to plan the date of your first injection. Now I am encouraging you to plan ahead for your last. I suggest you start to reduce your dose about three months before you stop treatment completely. Based on a two-year treatment period, that means you should prepare to reduce the dose twenty-one months after your first injection. Make a note of that date.

Step 2: Review your goals

Six months before you start to reduce the dose, review your goals. Have you achieved them – or are you well enough on track to achieving them to feel that you have succeeded? If not, what can you do to achieve success? Options include reviewing your diet (covered in the next step) or increasing the dose of medication, if there is scope to do so. If you have already achieved your goals, do you want to start reducing the dose early?

Step 3: Review your diet

At least three months before you start to reduce the dose, review your diet. Read Chapter 3 again and make sure you are maximising your chance of success for the remaining time you are on injections, and afterwards. Are you prioritising protein – using powder supplements if necessary? Are you including fibre from vegetables in your meals? Are you drinking enough water? Can you increase your intake of natural GLP-1 boosters (eggs, olive oil, lentils and nuts)? Have any highly refined carbohydrates sneaked back into your diet, such as sweet foods, cereals, white bread, pasta or rice? If so, try to replace them with protein and vegetables. Do you still experience cravings for certain foods? If so, list the foods and think of a plan to manage your cravings if they start to increase as you reduce the dose. This could include asking people close to you not to eat those foods in your presence, or offer them to you; making sure you do not have the foods in your house; and planning to go for a walk or engage in an enjoyable non-food activity when the cravings arise.

Step 4: Reduce your dose

Two weeks before you are due to reduce your dose, look at your diary. Does that date coincide with a big event, a time away from home, or any other situation that might make it harder for you to watch your diet? If so, consider delaying until after that event. When the time arrives, the easiest way to reduce the dose is to use the same injection pen and increase the number of days between injections. So instead of injecting every seven days, try increasing the interval by two days each time (to nine days, then eleven days). The rate of reduction is entirely up to you. If you don't feel any difference, you can increase the gap between injections each time. But if it is a struggle, you can take two or three injections with a nine-day gap before increasing the gap to eleven days. Once you are at eleven days, you can ask to be prescribed the next dose down and continue at the same frequency, reducing the dose every few injections. If you experience a raging appetite that you find very difficult to control, then revert to a weekly injection for a few weeks. Be guided by your body's reactions to the lower dose. Remember that if you use Mounjaro, increasing the time between injections is contrary to the manufacturer's recommendation, and so I recommend keeping the pen in the refrigerator.

Step 5: Feed your appetite

As you reduce the dose, your appetite will increase. This is where it is extremely important to stick to the dietary advice in Chapter 3. You will need to increase the volume of the food you eat, to avoid excessive hunger that could lead to cravings for unhealthy food. But make sure it is predominantly protein and vegetables that you increase, as this will have much less effect in increasing your weight than carbohydrates or excessive fats.

Step 6: Monitor your progress

In Chapter 7 I encouraged you to collect data, and this is an important time to do just that. Weigh yourself and/or measure your waist once a week. Accept that there will likely be a slight increase in both as you come off the injections, but if that increase risks undoing all the hard work you have done, do not delay before seeking further advice and potentially restarting or increasing treatment for a few weeks or months.

Step 7: Seek advice

Mounjaro and Wegovy are still relatively new treatments, and we are learning all the time about them, and especially about how to come off them. If you are finding it difficult to reduce the dose, despite making several attempts, then seek advice from your prescriber. If you have diabetes, adding metformin might help (or increase the dose, if you already take it). Maybe you have been able to reduce to a low dose every eleven or fourteen days, but cannot reduce any further. In that situation, your prescriber may be willing to continue your prescription at that low dose for a period of time, or you might consider purchasing some doses to enable a slower tailing-off of treatment.

Chapter 12
Life after injections

The unfortunate reality for many people is that once they stop weight-loss injections, the weight piles back on and they can end up back where they started. That is what many of the trials, funded by the drug manufacturers, show. One interpretation of this is that people need to stay on them for the long term (great news for the drug companies), but this is likely to be unaffordable for many people who are paying privately, or for health systems that pick up the bill. It is one of the reasons why, in the UK, the NHS limits the use of Wegovy to two years.

That's the bad news. The good news is that some people do manage to successfully come off the injections *and* keep their weight off. Throughout this book, I have aimed to provide you with all the information you need and the steps to take that will maximise your chances of keeping weight off in the long term. Steps, you will remember, *that start before your very first injection.* If you have been able to follow them, you will have changed your diet to prioritise protein, vegetables and healthy fats, and you will have banished sugary snacks and highly refined carbohydrates from the house. You will also have been doing strength training to build up your muscles and taken steps to manage stress and ensure good sleep. While on the injections, you will have been helped by the reduction in food noise, the loss of appetite, and even by nausea in managing your food intake. By using low doses and spacing out the injections, the aim is that you will have learned how to manage increased hunger and food noise by sticking to the same key principles. And sticking to those after your last injection is vital, to maximise your chances of long-term success.

So, as you come off injections, what can you do to help you stick to these principles? A key factor that helps people in this situation is support from family and friends. Now is the time to remind those around you that, even though you have lost a lot of weight, to keep it off going forward you will choose to follow a similar eating pattern, albeit with larger portions. Ask them to support you by not offering you foods that you are choosing to avoid – and if they live with you, ask them not to eat those foods in front of you. If you have addictive tendencies to certain foods, then now is the time to remind people these are the foods that you cannot eat. Even if you have managed to avoid these trigger foods while you were on the injections, now is not the time to be tempted by offers of biscuits or sweets. You can't just have one; you could very quickly find yourself back in a spiral of overeating and craving foods that will ensure you will regain weight. Your answer could be 'Thank you for the offer, but I cannot eat biscuits' or 'I am intolerant to biscuits and can't eat them'. You might not like to describe yourself as an addict, but many of us develop addiction-like relationships with certain UPFs, and to manage that addiction, we need to avoid those foods completely, just as an alcoholic needs to abstain completely from alcohol.

The changes you need to make to lose weight and then manage your weight need to be long-term changes. Day in, day out. Week in, week out – and of course year in, year out. Being addicted to certain foods can make that difficult, but even those who do not feel addicted to certain foods can find long-term change – any change – very difficult. Take one example. For many years, we have been led to believe that porridge is very healthy. As a cereal, it probably is the least bad one there is. But it is predominantly carbohydrate, and so risks promoting the obesity disease process described in Chapter 2. That is why I suggest switching away from all forms of cereal and to a breakfast based on protein and healthy fat, such as eggs or plain Greek yoghurt. I can recall a number of people who made this switch quite successfully, but three months later they were back on porridge. It wasn't that they didn't like their new breakfast; it was because their brains had been wired for decades to believe that porridge was their breakfast, and perhaps without consciously deciding to, they reverted to their decades-old habit. It really was a matter of 'old habits die hard'.

Intermittent fasting

Intermittent fasting first hit the headlines in 2013 when the late Dr Michael Mosley introduced us to the concept of the 5:2 diet in his book *The Fast Diet*.[61] Until then, I had associated fasting with religious practice, most obviously among Muslims who fast during daylight hours during the month of Ramadan. Fasting is also practised by many other faith groups, with claims that it helps cleanse the body and/or the spirit. It's fair to say that I was sceptical that fasting conferred any real benefits to physical health. But in his book Dr Mosley opened my eyes to the different ways in which fasting is beneficial to our physical health. One is that the body uses periods of fasting to undergo essential maintenance: fasting increases a process called autophagy, which literally means self-eating (that is, when the body rids itself of ageing and decaying cells). He also lists many other benefits of fasting, including increasing life expectancy, and improving heart

---

61 Mosley M and Spencer M (2014), *The Fast Diet: Revised and Updated: Lose weight, stay healthy, live longer.* Octopus Publishing Group.

and brain health. But the most striking impact of fasting is on the level of insulin in the bloodstream.

We learned in Chapter 2 how insulin levels increase when we eat a meal that contains carbohydrates, and that high insulin levels over time lead to excessive accumulation of fat in the liver and the pancreas, and this drives the development of obesity. Therefore, reducing carbohydrates reduces the insulin level in the blood. However, protein and – to a much lesser extent – fat also lead to some insulin being produced. In some people, this may be enough to stop them losing weight. However, when we fast, insulin levels fall dramatically. That is because there is no longer a steady stream of energy coming from our food, and so the body needs to access its stored energy. The first stores to be used are the glycogen (glucose) stores in the liver and muscles: when insulin levels fall, these are released into the blood. These are soon used up, and then the fat stored in the liver is used as energy. This use of fat stores in the liver is halted as soon as insulin levels rise again. Therefore, when we fast, insulin levels remain low, and the longer we fast, the longer our insulin levels remain low and the more our fat stores will be used up. Fasting is therefore remarkably effective at removing excess fat. The 5:2 diet is an approach whereby you eat normally for five days each week, but on two days, you 'fast'. Well, you don't fast completely; you are allowed one meal of about 500 calories. Michael Mosley used this approach to reverse his Type 2 diabetes, and many others have also found it successful.

I generally do not recommend fasting while on weight-loss injections, as appetite is reduced in any case and it is essential that you don't miss out on vital nutrients, especially protein. However, it can be very helpful to use fasting as you come off injections and afterwards. To my mind, the easiest form of fasting, also known as time-restricted eating, is to skip breakfast. Skipping breakfast is a great, easy way of fasting as you don't need to do any special planning for it; you just get up and go about your morning, skipping breakfast. This essentially creates a sixteen-hour fast each day. You can have an early lunch and an evening meal no later than 7 p.m. – you can even have a mid-afternoon snack if you wish. But then you eat nothing from 7 p.m. until at least 11 a.m. the next day. It is a relatively short fast, but a number of my patients have found it helpful when they wanted to lose more weight, or prevent weight gain. Some people are happy to miss breakfast every day, while others feel hungry on some mornings but skip breakfast on days when they do not.

So, if you're not usually hungry in the morning or you don't like breakfast, try skipping it.

There are other forms of intermittent fasting that are a bit more involved. Some people favour a twenty-four-hour fast once or twice a week. This is a variation on the 5:2 approach, but means that on a fasting day, you miss both breakfast and lunch and just eat an evening meal. Others routinely have just One Meal A Day (also called the OMAD approach) and feel perfectly well doing so. You might think you couldn't possibly manage missing one meal, let alone a whole day of meals, as you constantly feel so hungry. The reality is, that many people report they rarely feel hunger when they fast, and if they do, it soon passes, especially if they do something to take their mind off it. The reason is that hunger is largely driven by insulin, and if you are used to eating carbohydrates several times a day, you are keeping your blood insulin levels quite high, so you always feel hungry. Remember that during a fast, insulin levels *and* hunger are greatly reduced.

Fasting is not for everyone, and there is no one right way to do it, but if you wish to explore using fasting as part of your weight maintenance routine, I encourage you to find a plan that works well for you. It is essential to discuss with your doctor any changes to your medication that might be needed if you choose to fast, particularly if you take diabetes medications such as insulin or sulfonylurea tablets, or other tablets that need to be taken with food. Dr Jason Fung, a kidney specialist from Canada, is a leading expert on fasting, and his book *The Obesity Code* provides a wealth of information on the theory behind fasting and the practicalities of introducing it into your life.[62]

If, for whatever reason, you do not feel that fasting is for you, then I encourage you to use the evidence of its benefits and only to eat if you are hungry. Please ignore the instruction that you must not skip a meal. If on a particular day you get to lunchtime and you are really not hungry, then don't eat lunch. Or if you had a late, large lunch so that you're not hungry in the evening, skip your evening meal. If you meet a friend for coffee, remember that the coffee will fill your stomach and you really don't need to have something to eat with it. It is highly unlikely that our prehistoric ancestors sat down in their caves to eat three meals a day. In fact, the mechanisms that we have evolved to store excess energy as fat suggest quite the opposite. These mechanisms are a safety net, built up during periods of abundance for the lean times when there is no food available. The trouble is that for far too many of us, there is always too much food available – it's all feast and no famine. The more we can get back to a pattern of only eating when we are hungry, the better our bodies will be able to function, and the better metabolic health we will enjoy.

---

62 Fung J (2016), *The Obesity Code: Unlocking the secrets of weight loss*. New York: Greystone Books.

Getting back on track when you need to

Human nature being what it is, we can find ourselves going off track with our eating plan. It could be a holiday or a special occasion where you allow yourself to indulge in a food you have given up. Without the support of the injections, you could end up eating a lot more than you planned, and find that the return of food noise and food cravings are extremely difficult to resist. Others deviate from their new eating pattern because something else comes along that changes everything. I have had patients who had been doing really well, and then experienced a major 'life event', including the death of a spouse, a diagnosis of cancer, or loss of employment or housing. I do not need to explain how each of these can be such a shock to the system that they impact on a person's ability to stay on track with their new way of eating. While it might be possible to plan for a relapse for situations where you might be tempted in normal daily life, I am not sure that any of us can adequately plan for the impact of a major life event. Unfortunately, we all live with the possibility that something awful might happen to ourselves or to a loved one. So rather than trying to plan ahead, when this happens, the key is to accept that life has thrown a spanner in the works, manage the immediate impact on your eating pattern and your weight, and when the time is right, plan how you can get back on track.

So, what does this mean in practice? First, I encourage everyone in this situation to focus on everything they have achieved up until that point: all the weight they have lost, the reduction in their medications, the improvement in how they feel. Sometimes it is helpful to write these down in the form of a list. Then acknowledge that it is entirely natural to be thrown off course by what has happened. Be kind to yourself. Don't beat yourself up. However, if because of what has happened, your changed eating pattern or elevated stress level mean that your weight is on the increase, please seek advice about managing it. In my view, this is a situation where a return to a low dose of injections can be very helpful, at least in the short term. Once life begins to return to normal, you may well be able to come off them again.

In my experience, for most people in this situation, life does return to something more normal, and in each of the cases I mentioned earlier, the person was able to get back on track. But it will likely take time, and this is exactly the moment to seek the help of a close friend or a health professional who will provide you with emotional support as you work through the life event then begin to plan how to get back on track.

In Chapter 8, I touched on the importance of setting your goals in a way that gives you hope for a brighter future. If life has thrown a spanner in the works, it may be difficult to regain that sense of hope. If you do find yourself in this situation, I suggest you reread Chapter 8 and start again by setting yourself some new goals based on your changed situation and your new hopes for a healthier future.

Chapter 13

Future developments

New weight-loss medications

When a medication is first introduced to the market, it is covered by a patent which means the drug developer has sole rights to produce the medication. This enables the drug company to charge a premium price to recoup its – often significant – financial investment in the development, scientific evaluation and clinical trials of the drug before it can be authorised to be prescribed to patients. The patent generally lasts twenty years and is usually filed in the early stages of development. By the time the drug comes to market, the remaining life of the patent might be ten years or less. After the patent expires, other companies are able to produce the same molecule (known as a biosimilar or generic drug), and the price falls dramatically. Although it has only recently been introduced as a treatment for obesity, the patent for Wegovy is likely to expire in the UK in 2028, when much cheaper generic versions will become available. The patent for Mounjaro will continue until 2036.

So a significant future development is that, soon after 2028, cheaper versions of Wegovy will be available. Generic versions can be up to 60% cheaper than the original drug, and so it is likely that the NHS will provide it to larger numbers of people, easing the restrictions on who is eligible for it, and perhaps prescribing it for longer. It will also mean that the cost of purchasing the medication privately will become affordable to many more people.

In view of patent expiry dates, the pharmaceutical industry is geared up to a continuous production line of new drugs in development, known as a drug pipeline. This ensures that as the patent for one drug expires, the company can generate profits from a newer – and hopefully better – version. It will come as no surprise to learn that a number of companies have a range of new obesity drugs in their pipeline and these, when released, will offer new alternatives to the current treatments. Bear in mind, though, that as we discovered in Chapter 1, many obesity medications have come and gone, and most have either been ineffective or dangerous, so new drugs are not guaranteed to be any better than those currently available.

The first new drug likely to become available in the UK is Orforglipron, which is a tablet version of a GLP-1 medication that has to be taken every day. There is already a tablet version of Wegovy called Rybelsus. This is available as a treatment for Type 2 diabetes at a dose of 9 mg daily. It has been studied as a weight-loss drug at much higher doses, but this was associated with significant side effects in the vast majority of people taking it, so higher doses are not currently available. Orforglipron is manufactured by Eli Lilly (which also makes Mounjaro), and in clinical trials in people with obesity, it has resulted in up to a 12% weight loss.[63] It is likely to be available in the UK in 2026 and will be welcomed by those who do not wish to inject themselves.

Other drugs in development include those that, like Mounjaro, have more than one action. Retatrutide is produced by Eli Lilly and, like Mounjaro, has GLP-1 and GIP effects, and also activates glucagon receptors. Glucagon has the opposite effect to insulin and so promotes the burning of fat for energy, reduces fat storage, and increases satiety. Early trials suggest that retatrutide can cause up to a 24% weight loss. It should be available in the UK by 2027.[64] Survodutide is a GLP-1/glucagon agonist under development by Boehringer

---

[63] Wharton S, et al. 'Orforglipron, an oral small-molecule GLP-1 receptor agonist for obesity treatment.' *N. Engl. J. Med.*, 2025. doi:10.1056/NEJMoa2511774

[64] Jastreboff AM, et al. 'Triple-hormone receptor agonist Retatrutide for obesity—a Phase 2 trial.' *N. Engl. J. Med.*, 2023, 239: 514–26.

Ingelheim that should also be available in 2027. Amylin is a hormone that can promote weight loss by reducing appetite and food intake. It works by acting on brain regions that regulate appetite and satiety, and by slowing the emptying of the stomach. Cagrilinitide is a long-acting amylin analogue, which means it mimics the effects of amylin. Novo Nordisk is currently trialling a combination of cagrilinitide with Wegovy. Known as CagriSema, it is also likely to be available by 2027. At the time of writing, the price of these new drugs is unknown.

A different approach is employed by Rejuva. This is a gene therapy developed by Fractyl Health that is designed to programme the pancreas to produce GLP-1. This is at the very early stages of development, but something to look out for in years to come.

As we discussed in Chapter 7, anyone who loses a significant amount of weight will lose muscle as well as fat, and the use of weight-loss injections can lead to up to 40% of weight lost being muscle. This is why it's so important to ensure you include a good amount of protein in your diet and do regular strength-training exercises to minimise muscle loss. Meanwhile, companies are looking to adapt injections to try and minimise loss of muscle. One option being explored is to include a myostatin inhibitor. Myostatin is a protein that is produced by muscle cells to limit their growth to ensure muscles do not grow too large. In theory, adding a myostatin inhibitor to the injection should enable muscle to grow more and to offset the muscle lost because of the GLP-1 medication. However, there are concerns that while myostatin inhibitors increase muscle mass, the muscle tissue could be of lower quality so the muscles are still weak.

STNT-101 is a once daily tablet under development by Syntis Bio. The drug is broken down in the duodenum of the small intestine: it forms a thin coating along the inside of the duodenum that temporarily blocks the absorption of foods into the bloodstream. The nutrients then pass lower down in the small intestine where natural GLP-1 is produced. In theory, the combination of reduced absorption and increased GLP-1 aids weight loss, and this is currently being explored in early clinical trials.

While there are lots of new developments to look forward to in terms of medications to help people lose weight, please don't view these as even more of a wonder drug than Wegovy or Mounjaro. Remember, every single medication has side effects, and some of these drugs might have different effects to those we have become used to with Wegovy or Mounjaro. And even with these new medications, users will have to plan for when they come off them, which reiterates the need for people to address dietary changes as part of their weight-loss strategy, regardless of whether or not they are taking weight-loss medications.

Improving the food you eat

In this chapter on future developments, I feel it is important to talk about what else can be done to manage the obesity epidemic in the UK and many other countries. At the end of the day, obesity is a result of changes in our lifestyles that have taken place over the past few decades: we are less active now, and there has been a huge growth in UPFs, which are high in sugar and other refined carbohydrates: these now account for over 50% of food eaten in the UK.

In Chapter 3 I described how some campaigners liken UPFs to recreational drugs. I have to say, I agree. The way in which manufacturers have formulated foods so that they light up the happy parts of the brain to make us feel good when we eat them mean that they have more in common with recreational drugs than with real food. And yet, while governments around the world go to great lengths to outlaw recreational drugs, and (through taxation) to limit access to alcohol and tobacco products, many, including the UK government, have failed dismally to limit the harm done by UPFs. In recent years, the UK government has promised to limit TV advertising of UPFs, only for this plan to be ditched after lobbying from the food industry. In 2024, the new Labour government committed to introducing a ban on adverts for UPFs that targeted children: it is due to come into force in January 2026. This is to be welcomed, but there is still much more to be done – even the traffic light food labelling system, which is meant to inform people if foods are high in sugar, salt and fat, is only voluntary, which means that producers can choose to use it only on products that will show them in a good light.

Other countries have done much better. For many years, Chile has had mandatory labelling: a large black symbol must be placed prominently on the front of the pack of all products that are high in sugar, saturated fat, salt or calories. The symbols are hexagonal, to replicate the 'STOP' road sign. A product that is high in all four – sugar, salt, saturated fat and calories – must display four signs in a row, making the warning very prominent, just like the health warnings on packs of cigarettes. However, any product with just one of these warning signs is banned from schools, which has a direct impact on the health of children. One study showed that these actions have reduced the consumption of sugar by 10%, and saturated fat by 4%.[65] There is still some way

---

65 Tallie L, et al. 'Changes in food purchases after the Chilean policies on food labelling, marketing, and sales in schools: A before-and-after study.' *The Lancet Planetary Health*, 2021, 5: e526–33.

to go, but I hope that other countries will introduce similar regulations to guide people towards healthier food choices.

In the UK, we are seeing a rise in sales of butter and whole milk compared to margarine and low-fat milk:[66] there are early signs that consumers are turning away from the 'low-fat food is healthy' message that has been associated with the rise in UPFs in recent decades. This, together with a focus on restricting advertising, should lead to an improvement in the quality of foods eaten and should help reduce the number of people who develop obesity in the future.

Your healthier future

But what about you and your future? I really hope that reading this book has made you enthusiastic about making changes to your lifestyle that will allow you to lead a healthier life, long into old age, free of the physical health problems and the negative emotions associated with carrying excess weight. Whether or not you use weight-loss injections, making those changes will not be easy, but they will be so worth it.

---

66 https://www.ofimagazine.com/news/full-fat-milk-and-butter-sales-rise-in-uk-as-consumers-appetite-for-low-calorie-options-drops

A Guide to Weight Loss Injections

Obesity is a gradual process – it creeps up on you over many years. Reversing obesity and losing weight – and keeping the weight off – is likely to take some time to master. So, take things one stage at a time. First, focus on the changes you need to make before you start injections. Next, focus on the changes you need to make while you are on them. Finally, think about how you will come off them.

Perhaps you are reading this and feeling a sense of failure or resignation because you have tried every diet under the sun and none has worked. Remember that setbacks are normal, so please do not allow them to discourage you. Use them as an opportunity to revisit your goals and your hopes for what you can achieve when you have lost weight. Weight-loss injections provide a beacon of hope that you really can lose weight. They are a game-changer – they give you a break from constant hunger, food cravings and food noise while you reset your relationship with food. If you use them carefully and at low doses (if you can), in conjunction with diet changes and strength training, you can minimise their side effects and maximise your chance of success. I wish you all the very best on your weight-loss journey. I know you can do it!

Index

acenocoumarol 158
acid reflux 159, 161, 179
activity levels, historical changes 24–5
addiction
   food 30–4, 75, 125–6, 187–8, 212–13
   generally 124–5
age-related macular degeneration 141–2
ageing, muscle mass loss 140–1
alcohol
   GLP_{-1} agonists effect 124–5, 161
   reducing consumption 82–3
allergies 139
alternative diets 57
Alzheimer's disease 120
amphetamines 11–12
amylase 33, 39
amylin 226
anaesthesia 172
anxiety 189, 191–2

apoptosis 117
appetite
   amylin 226
   coming off injections 207–8
   dopamine 12
   effect of injections 83
   ghrelin 105
   GLP_{-1} agonists 104
   GLP_{-1} effect 14, 101–2
arteries, blood flow 117–18
atherosclerosis 45
Atkins diet 11
autophagy 214
avocados 65, 66

bananas 55, 74
Banting, William 10–11
bears 36
beer 82
Beeson, James 96, 99
Bennett, Steve 79–80
berries 75, 77, 81

beta cells, GLP$_{-1}$ effect 15
Bikman, Ben 165
bipolar disorder 188
bloating 134
blood–brain barrier 42
blood pressure 44, 45, 117–18, 138–9, 158, 178
blood tests, Type 2 diabetes diagnosis 43–4
body fat
    effect on blood glucose 40–1
    evolutionary function 35–7
    fasting effects 215
    GLP$_{-1}$ agonists effect 119
    inactivity 87
    insulin as storage hormone 40–1, 68
    leptin 42
    types 36
body mass index (BMI) 19–21, 149
brain
    GLP$_{-1}$ agonists effect 104, 118–19
    leptin 42–3
    obesity effects 48
    reward pathways 105, 124
bread 31–2, 33, 56, 61–2, 77–8, 79
breakfasts 76–7, 213, 216
breastfeeding 130
bupropion 203
burping 134
butter 61, 230
Byetta 13–14, 16, 123

cagrilinitide 226
CagriSema 226
calorie counting 67–70
cancer
    GLP$_{-1}$ agonists effect 121–2
    obesity effects 48, 121
    thyroid 5, 129
carb addiction 33
carbohydrates
    fruit and vegetables 54–5
    hunger 69
    reducing in diet 59–60, 61–2, 83
    restriction 57, 70–1
    starches 55–6, 61–2
    time of day 76
cardiovascular disease 45, 58, 63–4, 66, 117
cardiovascular outcomes trials (CVOTs) 116
carers support 6–7, 175–6
carnivore diet 57, 70
celebrations and sugar consumption 60
cereals 61–2, 76–7, 213
Chatterjee, Rangan 196
cheat days 176–7

cheese 66–7, 81
children
    BMI not used 19
    obesity levels 23
    weight loss injections 113–14
chocolate 31, 33
cholesterol 47, 87, 153
cholesterol levels 44
circadian rhythm 182–3
cirrhosis 45, 119
coconut 65
cognitive function 48, 188
comfort eating 138, 156
coming off injections 51, 199–209
compulsive eating 105
constipation 134, 135, 159
contraception 130, 136, 158, 173
cortisol 76, 183–4, 196
costs 110, 153, 200, 202
Couch to 5K 93–4
crackers 77, 81
cravings 34, 105, 169–70, 187–8, 206
cruises 177–8
cycling 28–9, 100
cytokines 48, 142

dairy products 65, 66–7
dehydration 132, 138–9, 161, 169, 171–2

dementia 48, 120–1
depression 48, 132, 157, 187, 189–91
desserts 81
dexfenfluramine 12
diabetes *see* Type 2 diabetes
diabetic eye disease (retinopathy) 130–1
diarrhoea 112, 133, 134, 136, 159
diet
    alternative diets 57
    avoid ultra-processed foods 60–1
    breakfasts 76–7, 213
    calorie counting 67–70
    carbohydrate restriction 57, 70–1, 83
    coming off injections 206
    cutting sugars 59–60, 71–3
    Eatwell Guide 52–4
    fats 63–7
    guidance for starting changes 70–83
    historical changes 25–6
    lunches 77–9
    'meat and two veg' 79–81
    Mediterranean 58
    protein 62–3
    reduce starches 61–2, 77–8
    snack reduction 73–5

before starting injections 155–7
UPF share 30, 228
dietary fats 63–7
digestive system
    energy requirements 69
    obesity problems 47
digoxin 136
doctor, involvement with treatment 108, 153, 157–8, 175, 208–9
dopamine 12, 32, 124, 138
dried fruit 55, 75
drinks
    alcohol 82–3
    cutting sugars 71–3
    fluid intake on injections 161, 169
    snacking 74
    sugar tax 34–5
drug pipeline 224
dulaglutide 114
duodenal ulcer disease 14

eating habits, permanent changes 51–2, 191
eating out 176
eating, time-restricted 216
Eatwell Guide 52–4
eggs 204
emotional eating 138, 156
endorphins 190

environment changes, historical 24–8
enzymes, pancreas 39
exenatide 16, 102, 122–3, 125
Exendin-4 16
exercise
    benefits 85
    cycling 100
    endorphins 190
    increasing 93–4, 156–7
    mental health 189–90
    strength training 95–100
    walking 86, 88–90, 96–7, 156–7, 185–6, 190
eyes, side effects 130–1, 141–2

fake products 109
family support 6–7, 175–6, 212–13
famine, history 2
fast-food, growth in availability 25–6, 27
fasting after coming off injections 214–18
fasting while on injections 161
fat, body *see* body fat
fat, dietary, addiction 33
fatty liver 44–5
Feltham, Sam 68–9
fenfluramine 12, 158
fertility 46–7, 122–3, 173

fibre 55, 56, 79–80, 160, 204, 206
fight-or-flight response 183–4
fish 65, 66, 78–9
food addiction 30–4, 75, 125–6, 187–8, 212–13
food deserts 26–7
food diaries 168, 169
food industry
   obesity effects 2
   snacks 73
   ultra-processed foods (UPFs) 29–30, 228
food labelling 229–30
food noise 105, 125–6, 169–70, 211–12
fructose 32
fruit
   carbohydrates 55
   cutting out of diet 60
   fructose 32
   smoothies 72
   snacking 74–5
Fung, Hason 217

gallstones 4, 47, 114, 131
gastric emptying 104
gastric inhibitory polypeptide (GIP) 16
gastroesophageal reflux disease (GERD) 47, 115
gastroparesis 4
gene therapy 226
ghrelin 105
Gila monsters 15–16, 102
GIP (gastric inhibitory polypeptide) receptors 106
gliclazide 178
glimepiride 178
GLP_{-1}, diet to maximise body's production 204, 206
GLP_{-1} agonists
   addictions effects 124–5
   brain benefits 120–1
   cancer effects 121–2
   effects on insulin 14–15
   fake products 110
   fertility effects 122–3
   first development 13, 102–3
   function in the body 104–5
   heart benefits 116–18
   interaction with other medication 136, 139, 157–8, 178–9
   kidney benefits 118
   liver benefits 118–19
   long-term treatment 199, 203
   sleep improvements 115
   see also injections; Mounjaro; side effects; Wegovy

GLP-1 (glucagon-like peptide 1)
    discovery 14, 102
    function in the body 101–2,
        117–18, 120
glucagon
    function in the body 225
    GLP-1 agonists 104
    GLP-1 effect 14
glucagon receptors 225
glucose
    alcohol 82
    effect of being overweight
        40–1
    function in the body 37
    GLP-1 agonists 104
    insulin control normal function
        39–40
glycogen
    effect of being overweight
        40–1
    function in the body 37–8
goal setting 146–52, 200, 205–6,
    220–1
gout 155, 179
GP, involvement with treatment
    108, 153, 157–8, 175, 208–9
grapes 55, 74
growth hormone 76
gut side effects 133–4, 158–9, 168,
    200

habits
    changing 213–14
    snacking 74
hair loss 137–8
hangovers 124, 161
HbA1c (glycated haemoglobin) 44,
    153
headaches 137
heart, GLP-1 agonists effect 116–18
heart attack 45
heart disease 63–4, 66, 67, 86, 133
heartburn 159, 179
Henry VIII 9
hibernation 36
high-fructose corn syrup (HFCS)
    32
hinges 98
history of obesity and treatments
    9–16
holidays 176–8
Holst, Jens Juul 14
hormones
    circadian rhythm 182–3
    disorders 46–7
    GLP-1 agonists 105
    time of day 76
    weight gain 37–43
HRT 158
hunger
    dose increases 169–70

fasting effects 217
ghrelin 105
GLP$_{-1}$ agonists 104, 105
hyperinsulinaemia 42
insulin 69
hunter-gatherers 36
hydration 161, 169
hyperinsulinaemia 41–2
hyperphagia 36
hypertension *see* blood pressure
hypoglycaemia 139, 158
hypotension 138–9
hypothalamus 42, 104, 190

ice cream 31, 33
illnesses while on injections 171–2
inactivity 87–8, 90–1
inflammation 48, 66, 118, 119, 120
injections
  coming off injections 51, 199–209
  day of the week 154–5, 162
  dose increases 111–12, 136–7, 164, 165, 167, 169–70
  dose reductions 206–7
  extending injection time 167–9, 206–7
  future generic versions 224
  method 110–11
  microdosing 112, 165–7

needle phobia 191–2
shortage of supply 201
switching drugs 170
time of day 159–60
tool for lifestyle changes 145–6, 167, 231
see also starting injections
insulin
  cortisol 184
  effect of being overweight 40
  fasting effects 215
  function in the body 37, 38–9, 68
  GLP$_{-1}$ agonists 104, 106
  GLP$_{-1}$ effect 14, 101
insulin/insulin resistance
  hunger 67–8
  hyperinsulinaemia 41–2
  mental health 48
  time of day 76
insulin resistance
  depression 187–8
  development due to weight 41
  fructose 32
  inactivity 87–8
  metabolic disorders 44–5
intermittent fasting 214–15
IVF treatments 122

joints, obesity problems 47

ketogenic diets 11, 57, 70
kidney disease 45, 133
kidneys, GLP$_{-1}$ agonists effect 118

labelling of foods 229–30
legumes 62
leptin 32
leptin/leptin resistance 42–3
levothyroxine 158, 178
life events, relapses 219–20
lifestyle changes
    advice during weight loss drugs usage 109
    coming off injections 205–6, 207–8
    injections as a tool 145–6, 167, 231
    permanent 51–2, 191, 211–12, 230–1
    setting goals 146–52, 200, 205–6, 220–1
    before starting injections 155–7
    see also diet
    stress 181–6
linseed 65
lipase 39
liraglutide 102–3, 122, 123
liver
    alcohol 82
    effect of being overweight 40–1
    GLP$_{-1}$ agonists effect 118–19
    glucose storage and function 38–9
    insulin function 39
    metabolic disorders 44–5
liver disease 133
long term effects 5
lunches 77–9

malnutrition, modern food system 2
margarine 61, 230
MASH (metabolic dysfunction-associated steatohepatitis) 45, 119
MASLD (metabolic dysfunction-associated steatotic liver disease) 44–5, 119
'meal deals' 26
meat 58, 65, 78
medication interactions with GLP$_{-1}$ agonists 136, 139, 157–8, 178–9
Mediterranean diet 58
medullary carcinoma 129
MEN2 (multiple endocrine neoplasia type 2) 129
mental health
    emotional eating 138, 156
    exercise 189–90
    GLP$_{-1}$ agonists 132, 138

obesity 48, 186–9
starting injections 157
stress 181–6, 189–91
wellbeing 193–4
metabolic acidosis 133
metabolic disorders 43–5
metabolic health and exercise 86–7
metformin 203, 204, 208
microdosing 112, 165–7
monounsaturated fat 64–5
mood disorders 48
moreish foods
addiction 30–1
moderation 66
Mosley, Michael 214, 215–16
Mounjaro
access to 107–10, 153–4
costs 110, 153, 200, 202
dose increases 111–12, 136–7, 164, 165, 167, 169–70
extending injection time 168, 206–7
function in the body 16
injection process 110–11
launch 105–6
NICE guidelines 3–4, 107–9
patent expiry 224
see also GLP-1 agonists
muscle mass building 95–6

muscle mass loss 5, 63, 83, 94–5, 140–1, 226–7
muscle-preserving antibodies 141, 226–7
muscle weight 19–20
musculoskeletal issues, obesity 47
myostatin inhibitors 226
Mysimba 203

NAION (non-arteritic anterior ischaemic optic neuropathy) 142
nature, spending time in 186, 190
nausea
alcohol 124
dehydration 132–3
minimising 134–5
starting injections 112, 134, 158–9
needle phobia 191–2
neurotransmitters 12, 48, 124
NHS
availability of weight loss drugs 107–9
costs of weight loss drugs 224
NICE (National Institute of Healthcare and Clinical Excellence), guidance on weight loss drugs 3, 107–10
nitric oxide (NO) 117

norepinephrine 12
nucleus accumbens (NAc) 124
nuts 64–5, 66

obesity
   cancer risk 48
   cardiovascular disease 45
   clinical definition 21–2
   common health problems 148
   costs to NHS 2–3
   definition 19–21
   digestive problems 47
   history 9–16
   hormonal disorders 46–7
   inflammation 48
   insulin function 40
   insulin resistance 41
   mental health 186–9
   metabolic disorders 43–5
   population levels 22–3
   preclinical 21
   respiratory issues 46
oesophageal reflux 47, 115, 179
oestrogen 46–7
oils 65
olives 66
omega 3 65
omega 6 65
One Meal A Day (OMAD approach) 217

Orforglipron 192, 224–5
Orlistat 13
osteoarthritis 47, 95
ovaries 122
Ozempic 16, 103

pancreas
   functions 39–40
   GLP_{-1} agonists 104, 106
   GLP_{-1} effect 14–15, 101
pancreatic disease 127
pancreatitis 4, 127, 171
Parkrun 93
pasta 56, 61–2, 81
pastry 61–2
patents 223
peptide YY 105
pharmaceutical industry, drug pipeline 224
phentermine 203
Phillips, Graham 166–7
pituitary gland 47
pizza 33–4
planks, straight-arm 99
plant-based diets 57–8
polycystic ovary syndrome (PCOS) 46, 122–3
polyunsaturated fat 65
porridge 56, 213
potatoes 55, 61–2, 81

prediabetes 44
pregnancy 122, 130, 173
private providers of weight loss drugs 109
proglucagon 102
protease 39
protein
  digestion requirements 69
  GLP$_{-1}$ production in body 204, 206
  meal focus 78–80
  muscles 63, 83, 141, 156
  preventing undernutrition 135
  priority in diet 62–3
  snacks 160–1
psyllium husk 135, 136, 159, 160
pulses 62

raisins 55, 75
Rejuva 226
respiratory issues 46
restaurants 176
retatrutide 225
retinopathy (diabetic eye disease) 130–1
rice 56, 61–2, 81
Rimonbant 12
Rollo, John 10
rosiglitazone 116
Rybelsus 225

salads 78
sandwiches 77–8
sarcopenia 140
satiety
  amylin 226
  GLP$_{-1}$ agonists 104
  GLP$_{-1}$ effect 15, 101, 106
  leptin 42–3
saturated fat 65–6
Saxenda 5, 103, 122
seeds 65
semaglutide 16, 103, 116
  see also Ozempic; Wegovy
serotonin 12
sex hormones 46–7, 122
shortage of supply 201
Sibitramine 12
side effects
  allergies 139
  carbohydrate restriction 70–1
  common list 4
  early usage 112
  eyes 130–1, 141–2
  food diaries 168, 169
  future drugs 227
  gallstones 4, 114, 131
  gut 133–4, 158–9
  hair loss 137–8
  headaches 137

historical weight loss medication 11, 12
hypoglycaemia 139
hypotension 138-9
mental health 132, 138
muscle mass loss 140-1
pancreatic disease 127
pre-existing conditions 132-3
pregnancy 130
reason for stopping injections 200, 202
reporting 137
starting injections 158-9
thyroid cancer 5, 129
vitamin deficiencies 139
sitting 87-8, 90-3
sleep apnoea 46, 115
sleep improvements 115, 179
sleep, prioritising 194-7
smoothies 72
snack reduction 73-5
snacking 156, 160-1
soups 78
special occasion events
   sugar consumption 60
   while on injections 173-4
spirits 82
squats 97-8
squirrels 35-6
standing 92, 93

starches
   conversion to glucose 33, 55-6
   reducing in diet 61-2, 77-8
starting injections
   health and medications review 157-8
   initial effects 112, 134, 158-9, 165-6
   lifestyle changes beforehand 155-7 *see also* diet
   measurements beforehand 153
   recording progress 162-4, 168
   setting goals 146-52, 200
   time of day 159-60
STNT-101 227
strength training 95-100
stress, effects and management 181-6, 189-91
stroke 45
strokes 120
sucrose 32
sugar
   addiction 32-3
   cutting out of diet 59-60, 71-3
   sugar rush 187-8
sugar tax 34-5
sulfonylurea 139, 178, 217
support network 6-7, 175-6, 212-13
surgery while on injections 172

survodutide 225–6
sweeteners 72

Taft, William 9
tapeworms 11
television viewing hours 88, 91
testosterone 46–7, 122, 123
thirst 161, 169
thyroid cancer 5, 129
thyroid hormone, thyrotoxicosis 11
thyrotoxicosis 11
time-restricted eating 216
tirzepatide *see* Mounjaro
topiramate 203
trans fats 66
triglycerides 44
Trulicity 114
Type 2 diabetes
    diagnosis 43–4
    GLP_{-1} agonists effect 5, 115
    medication interactions with GLP_{-1} agonists 139, 157–8, 178

UK, obesity levels 22–3
ulcers 14
ultra-processed foods (UPFs)
    addiction 30–4, 125–6
    advertising 228–9
    cognitive function 188
    consumption levels 29–30, 228
    diet restriction 60–1
    hunger 42
    taxation 34–5
undernutrition 134, 135, 139
urinary incontinence 48

vascular endothelial growth factor (VEGF1) 142
vasodilation 117
vegetables
    carbohydrates 55
    'meat and two veg' 78–81
    starches 62
Virta Health 203
vitamin deficiencies 139
vomiting 112, 133, 134, 159, 161

waist circumference 20, 87, 91–2
walkability of cities 28
walking 86, 88–90, 96–7, 156–7, 185–6, 190
warfarin 136
water retention 45
Wegovy
    access to 107–10, 153–4
    active ingredients 16
    costs 110, 153, 200, 202
    dose increases 111–12, 136–7, 164, 165, 167, 169–70

extending injection time 167–8, 206–7
function in the body 16, 104
injection process 110–11
launch 103
NICE guidelines 3, 107
patent expiry 223
see also GLP₋₁ agonists
weighing, recording progress 162–4
weight gain
  after finishing injections course 51, 202–4, 211
  hormones 37–43
  modern abundance of food 37
weight loss
  calorie restriction 69
  carbohydrate reduction 70
  exercise 85
  future medications and developments 223–8
  setting goals 146–52
  treatments history 9–16
wellbeing 193–4
wholegrain products 56
wine 82
work 'always on' 194–6

yoghurt 66–7, 77, 81

Zyban 203

RAISING READERS
Books Build Bright Futures

Dear Reader,

We'd love your attention for one more page to tell you about the crisis in children's reading, and what we can all do.

Studies have shown that reading for fun is the **single biggest predictor of a child's future life chances** – more than family circumstance, parents' educational background or income. It improves academic results, mental health, wealth, communication skills, ambition and happiness.[1]

The number of children reading for fun is in rapid decline. Young people have a lot of competition for their time. In 2024, 1 in 10 children and young people in the UK aged 5 to 18 did not own a single book at home.[2]

Hachette works extensively with schools, libraries and literacy charities, but here are some ways we can all raise more readers:

- Reading to children for just 10 minutes a day makes a difference
- Don't give up if children aren't regular readers – there will be books for them!
- Visit bookshops and libraries to get recommendations
- Encourage them to listen to audiobooks
- Support school libraries
- Give books as gifts

There's a lot more information about how to encourage children to read on our website: **www.RaisingReaders.co.uk**

Thank you for reading.

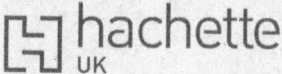

---

[1] OECD, '21st-Century Readers: Developing Literacy Skills in a Digital World', 2021, https://www.oecd.org/en/publications/21st-century-readers_a83d84cb-en.html

[2] National Literacy Trust, 'Book Ownership in 2024', November 2024, https://literacytrust.org.uk/research-services/research-reports/book-ownership-in-2024